Beginner Balance Exercises for Seniors

Prevent Falling Forever with 60+ Simple Home Exercises for Unshakeable Balance and Coordination

© **Copyright - All rights reserved.**

The content contained within this book may not be reproduced, duplicated or transmitted without direct written permission from the author or the publisher.

Under no circumstances will any blame or legal responsibility be held against the publisher, or author, for any damages, reparation, or monetary loss due to the information contained within this book, either directly or indirectly.

Legal Notice:

This book is copyright protected. It is only for personal use. You cannot amend, distribute, sell, use, quote or paraphrase any part, or the content within this book, without the consent of the author or publisher.

Disclaimer Notice:

Please note the information contained within this document is for educational and entertainment purposes only. All effort has been executed to present accurate, up to date, reliable, complete information. No warranties of any kind are declared or implied. Readers acknowledge that the author is not engaging in the rendering of legal, financial, medical or professional advice. The content within this book has been derived from various sources. Please consult a licensed professional before attempting any techniques outlined in this book.

By reading this document, the reader agrees that under no circumstances is the author responsible for any losses, direct or indirect, that are incurred as a result of the use of information contained within this document, including, but not limited to, errors, omissions, or inaccuracies.

Table of Contents

Introduction 1

Chapter One: Unsteady on Your Feet 5

   Why You're Losing your Balance 5

   Why It's Not Inevitable 11

   What You Can Do About It 14

Chapter Two: Busting Those Senior Fitness Myths 19

   Myth #1: Strength Training is too Dangerous For Me   20

   Myth #2: I'm Too Old to Exercise 21

   Myth #3: Strength Training Will Destroy My Joints   25

   Myth #4: Seniors should only exercise under the supervision of a physician 26

Chapter Three: How Balanced Are You? 29

   Static Tests 30

   Movement Tests 35

   The ABC Balance Confidence Scale 39

Chapter Four: Let's Make a Plan 42

   A Holistic Approach to Senior Fitness 42

   The Elements of a Comprehensive Balance Program   49

Chapter Five: The Warm Up 52

Dynamic vs Static Stretching ... 53
7 Dynamic Stretches Your Should Do ... 54
Chapter Six: Core Balance ... 61
Why You Need a Strong Core ... 61
10 Core Exercises ... 63
Chapter Seven: Phase One: Seated Exercises ... 69
12 General Purpose Exercises ... 70
3 Arthritis Friendly Exercises ... 76
Chapter Eight: Phase Two: Standing Exercises ... 78
12 General Purpose Exercises ... 79
3 Arthritis Friendly exercises ... 84
Chapter Nine: Phase Three: Vestibular Exercises 87
How the Vestibular System Works ... 87
The Cawthorne-Cooksey Vestibular Balance Exercises ... 89
Walking Balance Exercises ... 96
Obstacle Course ... 97
7 Walking Exercises ... 100
Chapter Ten: Putting It All Together ... 105
16 Week Training Program ... 109
Conclusion ... 138
References ... 140

~~$30~~ FREE BONUSES

Get Your Bonus Exercise Companion Videos
+ Printable Workout Tracker Sheets

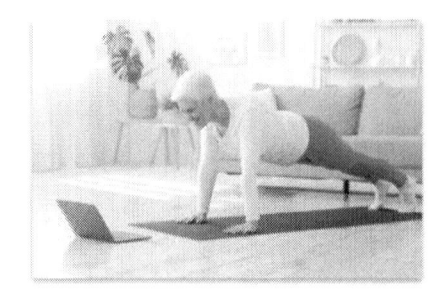

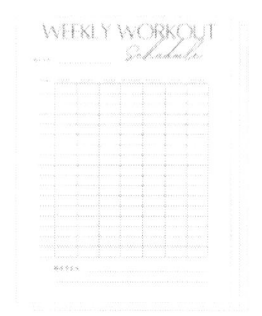

Scan QR code above to claim your free bonuses!

--- OR ---

visit https://bit.ly/3eaWvXF

Prepare to regain your rock-steady balance!

- ✓ Expert-guided exercise videos from the book so you can feel confident that you're doing them 100% right

- ✓ Tips & tricks to get the most out of your workout routines so you can reclaim your youthful strength & feel unshakeable

- ✓ Printable workout tracker sheets are included so you can guarantee that you're always progressing

Introduction

"Balance in the body is the foundation for balance in life."
Bks Iyengar

Balance isn't something we think about very much, and we often take it as a given until we start to lose it. When we're younger, some external influence often causes us to be unsteady on our feet - too much wine, being spun around, or a slippery surface underfoot. As we move into retirement and beyond, we start to gradually lose balance as result of muscle imbalances and tightness, deterioration of the vestibular system, reduction in bone density, and other natural causes of the aging process.

Loss of balance is one of the classic signs of aging, and people over sixty are often depicted as mobility challenged, bound to stumble and fall at the slightest obstacle. Aside from those caricatures, statistics and clinical studies suggest that loss of balance can be a serious issue and a leading cause of death in people aged 65 and over.

Although the situation may appear grim, loss of balance and mobility is not an inevitable consequence of aging. The ability to move your body freely through a range of motion without pain and without stumbling can be maintained and even enhanced by following daily exercise habits and controlling your weight.

That message was driven home to me on a trip to Taos, New Mexico, a few years back. There I learned on a tour that the original Pueblo dwellings had no doors. To get in and out, people had to climb up a ladder and then down another one. People of all ages, including the elderly, were able to scurry up and down these ladders with no trouble whatsoever.

Why were these people in their 60s, 70s, and 80s able to effortlessly get up and down these ladders when? According to traditional wisdom, they should have suffered the debilitating effects of aging on their balance and mobility.

The answer was obvious - they had maintained a lifetime of activity that allowed them to keep doing what they had always been doing. Of course, they were still affected by the natural decline in testosterone production and bone density that affects all humans, but their continued daily activity went a long way in reducing those deficits.

What can we draw from that experience?

Yes, we will experience weaker muscles and bones as we age. But that doesn't mean we are confined to a life full of imbalance and instability. By performing the right exercises, adopting an active lifestyle, and eating the foods that will enhance our well-being, we, too, can enjoy a life of both physical and mental balance.

This book has been designed to provide a bulletproof and comprehensive roadmap to becoming a physically confident, balanced senior. In the process, it will reject the conventional wisdom regarding seniors and balance and mobility issues. As a gym owner and personal trainer, I have seen and worked with too many elderly folks to buy into the inevitability of limited movement and unsteadiness as you age.

In the first three chapters, we'll redefine the expectations of balance and mobility in the aging population. You have probably heard of the phrase 'lowered expectations' for the younger generation. The same is true of seniors. Because elderly folks are expected to have poor balance, it's hardly surprising that we have such a huge problem with senior falls and other imbalance issues.

By challenging the myths and stereotypes about the physical abilities of seniors, we'll be able to set goals that will allow you to enjoy the freedom of movement you deserve. I'll then present you with some in-home testing you can do to determine your current balance level. That will give us a concrete level from which to set a goal.

In Chapter Four, we will take a step back to see how to balance training should fit into a holistic exercise program for seniors. While we won't go into detail on those other areas, I will provide some basic guidance to help you adopt a whole-of-life fitness plan.

Chapter Five is where the rubber hits the road. I'll show you how to ease into your balance exercise training with a warm-up program that will prepare both your aerobic and anaerobic systems for the exercises to follow.

The following chapters each focus on the next logical phase of a sound balance program:

- Core Training
- Seated Exercises
- Standing Exercises
- Vestibular Exercises

You won't find any exercise illustrations in these chapters. Instead, we have provided you with an accompanying PDF document that includes a video demonstration of every single exercise in this book. Watching a video is far more instructive than a picture or two!

Finally, we will put the exercises together in a 16-week progression of movements to take you from unsure on your feet to confidently mobile.

Reclaiming your balance is an empowering and liberating journey, but it's not one you have to do alone. Are you ready to reclaim your balance?

Let's do it together.

* * *

Chapter One:

Unsteady on Your Feet

"Balance is not something you find, it's something you create."

Jana Kingsford

Why You're Losing your Balance

You may be reading this book for a number of reasons.

Maybe you've reached a point of frustration after no longer being able to move as freely as you could just a few years ago. You might have experienced an unexpected fall and feel somewhat anxious about it happening again.

It could be that you're a caregiver for a beloved parent or relative and want a practical guide to help them improve their balance and mobility. Or, you could currently be moving with the aid of a walker and looking for exercises that can help you become more independent.

No matter your situation, and personal circumstances, my goal is to meet the expectations of each of these people. To do so, though, we must first understand the root causes behind the balance and mobility issues that negatively affect the quality of life of so many seniors.

According to the Vestibular Disorders Association, balance is *"the ability to maintain the body's center of mass over its base of support ... to allow humans to see clearly while moving, identify orientation with respect to gravity, determine direction and speed of movement, and make automatic postural adjustments to maintain posture and stability in various conditions and activities."*

We can distill this down to the ability to stay steady on your feet.

Many believe it's a natural skill that you either have or don't. However, it's not something we're born with. Babies are seriously lacking in balance for the first few months of their lives. But then, between the ages of four and six months, that changes as they learn to use and coordinate their muscles. That process evolves as they learn to crawl, walk and then run.

As a baby becomes a child and then a young adult, her balance and coordination improve. She's able to skateboard, dance, surf, and ski, But then, once she enters her fourth decade, changes start to occur that have an impact on her ability to maintain her balance. Here's a quick overview of the changes that directly relate to balance...

Bone Density Changes

From your fourth decade onward, you will start losing bone density. As a result, your bones will actually start to shrink. This will weaken your bones and make you more likely to suffer from a bone fracture if you slip, and fall.

As you age, your spinal vertebrae, sandwiched between your spinal discs, will contract. That's why you're now shorter than you were in your 20s. You've been losing half an inch every decade from 40 onwards. As your bones shrink in size, the sturdy foundation upon which your body relied for stability becomes less capable of keeping you upright, which reduces your overall balance.

Muscle Changes

From the age of 30, natural aging leads to a gradual loss of muscle tissue. As a result, you'll begin to slowly lose muscle, and find it harder to pack muscle even if you were doing the same workouts as before.

You've got two types of muscle fibers - fast twitch and slow twitch. You will lose both types, but the fast twitch fibers, which are responsible for quick, explosive movement, will go at a faster rate. As a result, your muscles will be slower to contract, affecting your reflexes, which are a crucial part of your balance.

So, how much muscle will you lose as a result of natural aging?

The average 75-year-old, who does nothing to reverse the process, will lose around 25 percent of the muscle mass they had at age 30. Muscle loss disproportionately affects the lower body. The large muscle groups of the lower body - the quadriceps, hamstrings, glutes, tibialis, and calves - are the very ones that are most involved in mobility and balance.

One other consequence of the reduction in muscle fiber number is that you will also lose strength. At the same time that you are losing muscle tissue, you're also experiencing a reduction in your number of motor neurons. These motor neurons are what control and drive muscle fiber activity. A 60-year-old will have lost 50 percent of the motor neurons they had at the age of 20.

The muscular system affects virtually every action that we take, so its weakening has profound effects on all areas of life. This weakness in the lower body muscles and motor neuron capacity is a major contributor to fall injuries among seniors. Its cumulative effect on body functioning shows itself as difficulty in performing everyday tasks, such as carrying groceries, walking up flights of stairs, or opening cans.

Hormonal Changes

Your hormones are the orchestra conductors of your body. They control everything that happens inside of you. A key class of hormones are the androgenic hormones that control male characteristics. While their key focus is on sexual functioning, they also regulate muscle mass and strength levels, as well as bone density and fat accumulation.

The most important muscle-building hormone is testosterone. Humans experience peak production of testosterone around the age of 25. From the age of 30 onward, you'll lose about one percent of your body's natural testosterone production every decade. This reduction in testosterone production is the main contributor to sarcopenia, the age-related loss of muscle tissue.

Even though it is a male sex hormone, testosterone is also important for women. That's because it is converted to estrogen (the female sex hormone) as well as promotes bone health, sex drive, and fertility.

Other hormones lower their production as we age. These include human growth hormone and melatonin. Even those hormones that maintain a constant level are affected by the diminished sensitivity of hormone receptors attached to cells. This makes them less effective.

Reduced levels of estrogen (the female sex hormone) speed up age-related bone loss. That's why women will lose bone density at a rate that is about 5 percent greater than men. It's also why senior women experience fall injuries more frequently than men.

Melatonin is often referred to as the sleep hormone. Its lowered levels contribute to the sleep problems that many older folks experience.

In men, the reduction of growth hormone combines with lower testosterone levels to further impact strength and muscle levels.

Brain & Nervous System Changes

Your brain will change more than any other part of your body as you age. It will actually begin to shrink from the age of 30 onward. This occurs faster in some parts of the brain than others.

The three areas that are most affected are:
- The prefrontal cortex
- The cerebellum
- The hippocampus

Every year after the age of 30, the neurons in your brain will become slightly smaller. They will also begin to retract their dendrites, with an accompanying reduction in the number of synapses between the brain cells. At the same time, the brain produces fewer new neurons, and the release of neurotransmitters, chemical messengers, like dopamine and serotonin, slows down.

While muscle and bone density changes affect your body's capacity to keep balance, the slow process of cognitive decline affects your brain's ability to maintain balance altogether.

Decline in various brain circuits, and your vestibular system has a cumulative effect, which leads to our reflexes slowing down, a higher struggle to maintain balance, and effectively cordinate our movements and adapt based on our current environment.

Body Composition Changes

Hand in hand with the age-related loss of muscle tissue, many people experience an increase in their levels of body fat. Your metabolism will slow down every year after the age of 30. That makes it very difficult for a person in his 60s, even if he is eating the same foods as he did in his 30s, to maintain the same weight. Even though he's taking in the same amount of calories, he will be expending less energy, resulting in caloric excess. That excess will be stored as body fat.

Largely due to the slowing of the metabolism, the average person will gain a pound of fat every year. That means that most 60-year-olds are carting around 30 more pounds than when they were 30!

The increase in body fat percentage means your muscles, and bones, which are already strained by their decline in mass, and density, have to carry around and balance even more weight, which exacerbates balance issues.

Why It's Not Inevitable

Having read about all of the physiological changes that occur as we age, you might conclude that loss of balance, unsteadiness on your feet and impaired mobility are an inevitable, unavoidable consequence of aging.

Don't believe it.

There are too many examples of people in their sixties, seventies, eighties and beyond who are agile, mobile and physically strong for that to be the case. I have worked with many of them in my role as a personal fitness trainer. The common thread between these folks is that they were all physically active.

I've already mentioned that falls are the leading cause of death for people over the age of 65. But when we dig a little deeper, we discover that 'age' is not the cause of these injuries. According to the Centers for Disease Control and Prevention, fall injuries in the senior population are the result of:

- Lower body weakness
- A sedentary lifestyle
- Improper gait
- Foot problems [1]

None of these conditions are inevitable. They are the result of a decreased level of activity and the incremental effects of poor posture and gait habits. On the other hand, those people who have been able to stay steady on their feet as they age have, as a general rule, followed an exercise program that strengthens their muscles and bones, improves their agility and mobility, and gives them the confidence to move without fear.

Moving without fear is a huge factor in achieving physical balance. The fear of suffering a fall injury is very real among seniors. You may be experiencing it yourself, especially if you've already had a nasty fall accident. That fear of falling can affect the way a person moves. And ironically, it can make them more likely to suffer a fall injury in the future.

Some interesting research was published in the *Journal of the American Geriatrics Society* in 2002 on the relationship between falling and the fear of falling. The researchers found that seniors who had not actually suffered a fall injury but who had a fear of falling were more likely to suffer from a fall injury despite the fact that they adjusted their lifestyle to lessen their likelihood of a fall! [2]

So, why would these people be more likely to fall even though they are cutting back on potentially dangerous activities? Well, it turns out that the fear of falling prevents people from doing the very things that they should be doing to become more mobile and steadier on their feet. Rather than further restricting their movements, they need to increase their activity levels.

The fear of falling has resulted in another common feature among the elderly; the senior shuffle. This movement is typified by a stuttering, cautious shuffling motion with small strides, a stiff upper body, and a very slow rate of advance.

Studies indicate that the senior shuffle is more likely to have an emotional rather than a physical cause. Research published in the journal *Gait Posture* in February 2005 concluded that …

"Gait changes in older adults who walk with fear may be an appropriate response to unsteadiness, are likely a marker of underlying pathology, and are not simply a physiological or psychological consequence of normal aging." [3]

In other words, old people don't do the senior shuffle because they are old. They do it because they are afraid of falling. It is not due to the natural consequence of aging.

If you've ever had to walk on ice, you know that it's only natural to adjust your gait to the conditions underfoot. The problem with many seniors is that they consider every underfoot condition to be risky and, so, move as if they are walking on ice all the time.

Unfortunately, the senior shuffle actually makes a person more likely to have a fall. When you walk this way, you are not moving your lower body muscles the way they were designed to facilitate advanced movement. The ankles hardly move and so become even less agile.

As a consequence of the almost imperceptible knee movement, the natural hip engagement of proper gait movement is severely restricted. The resulting hip stiffness, quadriceps tightness, and overall mobility reduction can increase your chances of injury.

Weaker hips, tighter thighs, and less mobile ankles are not what you want. That's why achieving greater physical balance as a senior needs to begin in your mind.

What You Can Do About It

You will never get your balance back until you master the fear of falling. As with most things, the root of this fear for many lies in the unknown.

Children tumble all the time, but, as adults, it hardly ever happens.

So, it's not surprising that the fear of falling can be a real worry. We conjure up images in our minds of broken bones, torn flesh, and excruciating pain. As we've seen, that fear can cause people to stiffen up their bodies and move in a very unnatural and unsafe way.

One sound strategy is to try and change your mindset. Examine your anxiety, and fear, are they based in reality? Although there's a small chance of getting injured, its relatively low, especially if you are mindful of your steps, and physically active for your age. Notice how fear has you in its grip, and makes you afraid to meaningfully live out your golden years.

Beliefs, especially irrational fears, can be powerful, and may have been formed for many years. To combat them effectively, you should catch yourself whenever you have such thoughts, and imagine nightmares of falling, and explain to yourself why they are not rooted in reality. For example, you can take a few slow breaths before a walk, and remind yourself that you will be fine before starting.

Not only is the chance of falling low, but it will get even lower once you take charge by embracing a holistic exercise program to improve not only your ability to balance but to make your entire body stronger, more muscular, and more robust.

Remind yourself of your childhood years, your bones may not be as sturdy as they were before, but a fall didn't have to be the end of the world. You can practice falling the right way.

After all, it's not falling that is the problem. It's the way the body reacts to the challenge of falling. As a personal trainer who works with seniors, I teach my clients how to fall safely. This not only prepares them to protect their body if they do suffer a tumble, it also goes a long way to helping them overcome the fear of falling.

> *Elliot's Story*
>
> At the age of 95, UK pensioner Elliot Royce reckoned that he'd fallen around 15,000 times in the previous 10 years. And every time it was on purpose.
>
> After suffering a serious fall in his early 80's, Elliot's family encouraged him to move into an assisted care facility. But, being the independent minded man that he was, Elliot sought a way to prove that he could still live by himself. He decided to tackle the fall issue head on by practicing safe falling.
>
> Elliot looked all over his local area for someone who could teach him how to fall safely. Unable to find anyone, he took to the internet. There he came across a course that was being run in Hawaii. So the determined nonagenarian purchased a ticket and headed to Honolulu. There he learned the 'twist-bend-roll' fall method.
>
> Upon his return to the UK, Elliot began a daily routine of safe falling, landing on an air mattress. As well as acquiring a reflexive safe falling method, he has been able to learn how to safely get up from the floor - something which many older people have great difficulty with.

> After getting exposure in the local press, Elliot began touring care homes and retirement villages to teach other elderly folk how to fall safely. He told his audiences …
>
> *Once you start to fall, you don't have time to think about what you do. You're going to have about one second to figure it out, so you better have some plans!*
>
> Six steps to falling safely …
>
> 1. Tuck your chin in.
> 2. Turn your head to the side.
> 3. Put your arms in front of your head.
> 4. Twist your body so you land on your side.
> 5. Bend your legs,
> 6. When you hit the floor, begin to roll to reduce impact.
>
> To make these reactions intensive, practice falling five times per day.

know you've bought this book, and that's a great start. But, the reality is that the vast majority of people who read exercise guides like this end up doing absolutely nothing about it.

Don't be one of them. Take action to change your circumstaces.

Your body deserves to be freed from the mental and physical restrictions that are imposed on it through your lack of proactive movement.

The 52 beginner balance exercises for seniors that are presented in this book will provide you with tools to ease into a progressive program to reclaim the independence and confidence that you once had. But it's up to you to make use of them.

Key Point Summary:

- As we age, we lose bone mass and muscle tissue, our hormones change, brain neurons become smaller and our metabolism slows.
- Despite these changes, balance issues are not inevitable.
- Fall injuries are caused by lower body weakness, a sedentary lifestyle, improper gait and foot problems.

In the next chapter, we'll reveal the truth about some persistent senior balance and fitness myths.

* * *

Chapter Two:

Busting Those Senior Fitness Myths

"The naive person believes every word, but the shrewd one ponders each step."

Proverbs 14:15

The fitness industry is full of lies, half-facts, and deliberate misinformation.

That might sound like a bold claim, but having been in the fitness industry for the bulk of the last four decades, however, I can tell you that it is a fact. It should come as no surprise, then, that much of what we think we know about senior fitness is widely inaccurate, preached by people who have a personal interest in spreading misinformation.

I could write a separate book about fitness myths, but, for our purpose, four prominent myths about seniors and exercise will do the trick nicely.

Myth #1: Strength Training is too Dangerous For Me

This myth is not as persistent as it used to be. However, some senior websites are still advising people not to do any type of strength training exercises. I notice, however, that they never provide any accompanying research to support their advice.

That's because the research to support not strength training in old age does not exist. In contrast, there is voluminous evidence to show that strength training is, in fact, one of the best things seniors can do to improve their quality of life.

Studies conducted over the past decade have shown that regular strength training can significantly reduce the symptoms of the following age-related conditions:

- Arthritis
- Poor balance
- Diabetes
- Osteoporosis
- Obesity
- Back pain
- Breathing problems
- Depression
- Dementia

In addition to making you less likely to suffer from these and other health conditions, strength training will make you far more functional in your everyday tasks.

A meta-study out of the Department of Occupational Therapy at Indiana University-Purdue University Indianapolis analyzed 121 trials involving 6,700 study participants between the ages of 60 and 80. The researchers concluded that seniors who participated in strength training workouts two to three times per week consistently outperformed those who didn't work on common daily movements. [4]

In terms of being dangerous, strength training is completely safe if it is done properly. Strength training will make your body stronger and safer if you learn and use the proper movement patterns, resistance level appropriate to your current fitness level, and the right programming.

Strength training that works all of the body's major muscle groups should be at the center of the prescription for healthy aging. But it should not be done to exclude cardiovascular training, such as walking, running, biking, etc. They have slightly different health benefits, but work together to improve your balance and overall fitness level.

Myth #2: I'm Too Old to Exercise

Your body is designed to move, so you begin to feel stiff and full of soreness and aches whenever you stop going for your daily walk, do some form of stretching, and stay immobile for extended periods. Your body may have lost some of its total functioning capacity in terms of bone density and muscle mass, but you are still very capable of exercising.

As we found out in the last chapter, inactivity is a major contributor to mobility, imbalance, and other physical problems that affect seniors. The only solution is to become physical activity.

Sedentary seniors are more than twice as likely to have cardiac health problems. They are also more likely to take multiple medications. The key is to find exercise appropriate to your abilities and make gradual but consistent progression. Swimming, for example, represents a low-impact way to move your muscles and get your heart pumping.

There's a wealth of studies proving conclusively that exercise is beneficial - and not harmful - for the elderly. One example is a 1999 study that involved 215 older folks who were assigned to either a home-based resistance exercise training group or a waiting list control group. The exercise group followed a videotaped exercise routine with resistance bands. The workouts were done three times per week for six months.

The exercise group had significant lower extremity strength improvements of 6% to 12%, a 20% improvement in tandem gait, and a 15% to 18% reduction in physical and overall disability at the 6-month follow-up. No adverse health effects were encountered. They also had significant improvement in their balance and mobility. [5]

A number of studies have also shown that even seniors with existing disease conditions, orthopedic impairment, and severe muscle atrophy are fully capable of participating in strengthening workouts if the program is prescribed by a therapist, doctor, or fitness professional. [6]

The research also makes it clear that age-related muscle strength and mass decrease can be offset by a regular strength training program. By combining strength training with exercises focused on improving balance, mobility, and flexibility, such as the 52 exercises that we will cover in the following chapters, a person can significantly decrease their risk of a fall while also increasing her functional independence so that she can carry out everyday tasks with confidence.

It may feel impossible and disheartening if you've been immobile for a while, and a brisk walk leaves you gasping for air, but you shouldn't get discouraged. Your body has a fascinating ability to adapt to the physical demands you put on it, and it will require a bit of time to get used to it.

When it comes to exercise, the human body follows the SAID principle. SAID stands for specific adaptation to imposed demands. When we place a demand on our body through repeated exercise, the body will adapt by becoming stronger in order to meet that challenge in the future. That will happen whether you're nine or ninety!

Renee's Reluctance

In her younger days, Renee was pretty active. She played tennis twice a week right into her fifties and even had a stint at the gym for a few years. By 70, though, all of that was long gone. She just didn't have the energy for exercise anymore. Besides, her bones and joints had become creaky, and she had a constant ache in her lower back. She figured that she was just too old for exercise.

Renee was an avid gardener. Her flower bed was her happy place. One day she was getting up from weeding around her prize white roses when she lost her balance and fell. Her head caught the edge of her garden shovel, and her right hip took the brunt of the impact with the ground. She ended up with seven stitches for the cut on the back of her head and a fractured hip.

The physical damage eventually healed with no lasting effects. But the psychological effects of Renee's accident were more long-term. A fear of falling again caused her to go into herself. She no longer gardened, replacing that special time in the dirt with hours of scrolling through Instagram looking at other people's gardens!

Renee's entire way of standing and walking also changed. She adopted the classic senior shuffle, becoming more stooped over with rounded shoulders and a downward stare. Needless to say, as a result of her fall, her quality of life was diminished.

As a personal trainer, I was introduced to Renee as the result of a personal trainer gift voucher from her son and daughter-in-law. To say that she was reluctant to do any type of balance exercise during our first consultation is an understatement. But we persevered, and I was able to gradually introduce the very same sitting balance exercises covered in Chapter 7 of this book. Within a month, Renee regained some of her confidence, and we were able to move on to the standing exercises.

Renee is now closing in on 80 years of age. Not only is she back out in the garden twice per week, but she's also joined a senior Pickleball club and does strength training every morning with a set of dumbbells that she keeps by her bed. She says that her new active routine has given her back the vitality and enjoyment that she thought was gone forever.

Myth #3: Strength Training Will Destroy My Joints

This myth is a hangover from the outdated orthopedic doctrine of times gone by. The reality is that the opposite is true. Strength training provides a whole host of benefits to the joints.

For people with osteoarthritis and similar conditions, it will decrease pain, preserve function, maintain mobility, decrease inflammation, increase muscle and bone mass around the affected joints and help to preserve a person's self-efficacy and independence.

To maintain healthy joints, you need an ample supply of oxygen and nutrients to help them regenerate and grow stronger. There's nothing like aerobic and strength training to promote healthy inflammation and improve circulation toward them.

Of course, strength training will not cure conditions like arthritis. People with advanced bone-on-bone disease will require new joints or similar intensive measures. But after they've had the procedure, I recommend beginning a supervised strength training program. It will make the joints and supporting muscles stronger and more mobile. [7]

Myth #4: Seniors should only exercise under the supervision of a physician

While it is good to be cautious regarding exercise, the belief that seniors are too frail to work out has led to the contention that they can only begin an exercise program after getting the go-ahead from a physician. Too often, this becomes a self-imposed barrier that stops the person from ever starting.

The reality is that if you do not have a diagnosed disease or any symptoms of one, you don't have to wait for a doctor's approval before beginning an exercise program. The only exception would be if you were about to embark on a high-intensity exercise regime, which I do not recommend for most seniors.

Of course, nothing is stopping you from getting approval from your doctor. Doing so can instill a sense of security and confidence. My point here is that it is not mandatory unless you suffer from a disease.

If you are joining a gym or working with a personal fitness trainer, you should expect that they will analyze your medical history and, if appropriate, direct you to a physician for informed consent before beginning the exercise program.

Pickleball anybody?

Pickleball.

Strange name for a game!

But that hasn't stopped it becoming one of the fastest growing sports in the United States. Pickleball courts can be seen in driveways and public venues all over the country. Some of the most popular members of communities up and down the nation to take up the pickleball habit are people over the age of 60.

The combination of fun, moderate intensity exercise, social camaraderie and relatively low skill entry level makes pickleball a great choice for the silver haired set.

> In addition to its cardiovascular benefits, pickleball provides a relatively joint friendly way to improve agility, proprioception (that's your awareness of what your body is doing), balance and mobility.
>
> Pickleball and healthy aging go together. The benefits that you get from this sport in terms of enhanced cardiovascular and anaerobic fitness are tremendous. Not to be overlooked are the social benefits of playing this fun game and the friendships and associations that stem from it.

Key Point Summary:

- Strength training is not dangerous for seniors. It is, in fact, one of the best things that older folks can do.
- Exercise has no age limits.
- Strength training will make your joints and supporting muscles stronger and more mobile.

In the next chapter, we'll present you with a series of tests to help you determine your balance starting point.

* * *

Chapter Three:

How Balanced Are You?

"You can't help getting older, but you don't have to get old."

George Burns

In order to improve your balance, you need to know what your balance is like right now. That will provide you with a baseline from which you can assess your improvement. In this chapter, I'll present some simple self assessment balance tests that you can do right now in the comfort of your home.

In these tests, you will be generating some facts and figures that need to be recorded for future testing comparison. I recommend getting a notebook where you can record your results for each test.

If possible, have a friend on hand to time you during the exercises.

Static Tests

These tests get progressively more difficult. If you are unable to complete a test, stop at that point and go onto the movement tests.

Standing Cushion Test

Length of Test: 60 seconds

Difficulty level: low

1. Place a chair cushion on the floor with a chair alongside that you can grab for balance if needed.
2. Stand on the cushion with your feet shoulder width apart. Stand up nice and tall, with your shoulders back. Clasp your hands together in front of your body.
3. Stay in this relaxed position for 60 seconds.
4. Make a note of whether you are able to achieve a 60 second position without holding the chair for balance. If you can't, then record how many seconds you were able to stay in position.

Standing Feet Together Test

Length of Test: 30 seconds

Difficulty level: high

1. Stand on the floor (no pillow) with your feet together and hands clasped in front of your body.
2. Stay in this relaxed position for 60 seconds.

3. Make a note of whether you are able to achieve a 60 second position without holding the chair for balance. If you can't, then record how many seconds you were able to stay in position and how many times you needed support.

Standing Feet Together Test (Eyes Closed)

Length of Test: 60 seconds

Difficulty level: medium

1. Stand on the floor with your feet together and hands clasped in front of your body. Now close your eyes and keep them closed for the entire test.
2. Stay in this relaxed position for 60 seconds.
3. Make a note of whether you are able to achieve a 60 second position without holding the chair for balance. If you can't, then record how many seconds you were able to stay in position and how many times you needed support.

Semi-Tandem Stance Test

Length of Test: 60 seconds

Difficulty level: medium

1. Stand with your right foot slightly in front of your left foot, so that they are side by side, with the big toe of the left foot is in the arch of the right foot.
2. Stand nice and tall, with your shoulders back and down.

3. Stay in this position for 60 seconds, being sure to maintain an upright posture.

4. Make a note of whether you are able to achieve a 60 second position without holding the chair for balance. If you can't, then record how many seconds you were able to stay in position and how many times you needed support.

5. Repeat with the left foot forward.

Note: Due to different levels of mobility, and muscles imbalances, it is quite common for one side to be less balanced than the other.

Tandem Stance Test

Length of Test: 60 seconds each leg

Difficulty level: high-medium

1. Place your right foot directly in front of the left foot, with even weight on both feet. Feel free to hold a chair to get into position.

2. Stand nice and tall, with your shoulders back and down.

3. Stay in this position for 60 seconds, being sure to maintain an upright posture.

4. Make a note of whether you are able to achieve a 60 second position without holding the chair for balance. If you can't, then record how many seconds you were able to stay in position and how many times you needed support.

5. Repeat with the left foot forward.

Single Leg Test

Length of Test: 60 seconds each leg

Difficulty level: high

1. Make sure there is a chair alongside for support during this exercise.
2. Stand in an upright position with your hands clasped in front of your body and feet about shoulder width apart. Now bend your right knee to bring the foot off the floor.
3. Maintaining an upright position, hold the one legged position. Try to maintain the position for 60 seconds.
4. Make a note of whether you are able to achieve a 60 second position without holding the chair for balance. If you can't, record how many seconds you were able to stay in position and how many times you needed support.
5. Repeat with the left foot elevated.

Single Leg Test With Arm Curls

Length of Test: 30 seconds each leg

Difficulty level: high

1. Make sure there is a chair alongside for support during this exercise.
2. Stand in an upright position with your hands clasped in front of your body and feet about shoulder width

apart. Now bend your right knee to bring the foot off the floor.

3. Maintaining an upright position, hold the one legged position. Now begin performing arm curls by curling your arms up to shoulder level and then back down.

4. Make a note of whether you are able to achieve a 30 second position without holding the chair for balance. If you can't, then record how many seconds you were able to stay in position and how many times you needed support.

5. Repeat with the left foot elevated.

Why We Fall

The five key risk factors for a fall have been identified as:

1. Poor eyesight that prevents people from seeing obstacles that are in their way.

2. Medications, whether prescription or over-the-counter, that produce such side effects as dizziness and lethargy. The worst medications in this regard are antidepressants, sedatives and tranquilizers.

3. Improper footwear or foot pain that prevents the brain receiving the needed sensory feedback to negotiate the terrain.

4. Environmental hazards, the most common of which are dim lighting, loose carpeting, uneven steps, spilled liquids and electrical cords.
5. Weakness in the quadriceps, glutes, hamstrings and core.
6. Weak bones, as a result of a lack of resistance movement, and vitamin and mineral deficiencies, like a deficiency in magnesium, zinc, calcium, and vitamin D.

Movement Tests

TUG Test

TUG stands for 'time to get up and go'. You'll need another person to time you during the test.

To prepare to do the test, put an item, such as a set of car keys or a book on the floor ten feet (3 meters) in front of a chair. Your partner should be holding a stopwatch. Their job is to time how long it takes you to get up from the chair, walk around the object and return to the chair. They should press the stop button on the timer when your butt touches the seat of their chair.

Sit nice and tall in the chair. When your partner says 'Go, get out of the chair and walk around the object, returning to the chair. Do this as quickly, but as safely, as you can.

Your partner should now record the time you took to complete the task. They should also not whether you needed to push off the seat handles to get up.

I recommend doing this test every four weeks. For consistency's sake, you should use the same chair every time you do the test. If you can reduce your time and get up without the assistance of the handles, this is a great sign of progress.

Five Time Sit to Stand Test

This test involves going from sitting to standing five times in a chair. You can use a chair with an armrest for extra support if you wish. This is another timed test, so you'll need a partner with a stopwatch in hand.

This test is not a race. Simply get up and down safely and comfortably as you normally would five times in a row. When you come up from the seated position, go all the way to a standing position. Then go all the way back to a seated position. Control the motion throughout. If you have to plonk down on the chair, stop and only count the time and number of repetitions completed under control.

Your partner should record the time it took to complete the five repetitions. They should also note whether you had to use the armrests, whether you appeared to lose your balance or muscle control, and any other things they feel are important.

Six Minute Walk Test

This test involves walking non-stop for six minutes. You should only do the test if your current condition will allow you to do so. If you use a cane or a walker, that is fine. The test can be done in any area with a hundred feet (33 meters) of flat walking space. [8]

Begin by marking out a hundred feet of flat walking space. Then stand on the start line. Your partner will tell you to begin and you simply walk normally up and down the hundred foot distance for a total of six minutes. Your partner should not talk to you during the time of the test.

Maintain your normal walking pace during the test. If you feel tired, you can lean against a wall to rest until you feel ready to continue. Stop the test immediately if you feel chest pain or experience difficulty breathing.

Your partner should be keeping a record of how many times you cover the hundred foot distance. They should instruct you to stop the second six minutes is up. They should then place a marker at the point you got to. You can then sit down and recover.

Your partner needs to calculate your total distance by adding the number of complete lengths and then measuring the partial distance covered on the last lap. Add this to give a final total. They should then record this total distance, along with any notes about whether you had to rest, lost your balance or veered off track.

Your Balance Systems

Your ability to remain steady on your feet is the result of three of your body's systems working seamlessly together. These are the visual, vestibular, and proprioceptive systems.

The visual system sends messages from the eyes to the brain to tell it how to react to the environment. That's why it's harder to stand up with your eyes closed; the visual cues are absent, throwing off your balance equilibrium.

The vestibular system is centered around the inner ear. It comprises a series of semicircular canals and receptors that determine the angle of the body to provide awareness of motion and equilibrium. When you go on a boat, your vestibular system will take some time to adapt to the oscillation of the waves. Until it does, you will experience motion sickness.

The proprioceptive system governs your body's awareness of the positioning of your arms and legs. Proprioceptive sensors are located in your muscles, joints, and skin to direct the body to adjust to the type of surface that you are standing or sitting on.

The ABC Balance Confidence Scale

The Activities Specific Balance (ABC) Balance Confidence Scale is a self assessment that involves rating your confidence level to do 16 different activities between 0%, where you have no confidence at all, and 100% where you are absolutely confident. [9]

Score yourself between 0 and 100% on the following activities without the use of a walking aid:

1) Walk around the house?
2) Walk up or down stairs?
3) Bend over & pick up a slipper from the floor?
4) Reach for an item on a shelf at eye level?
5) Stand on tiptoes & reach for an item above your head?
6) Stand on a chair and reach for something?
7) Sweep the floor?
8) Walk outside the house to a parked car?
9) Get into or out of a car?
10) Walk across a parking lot to a mall?
11) Walk up or down a ramp?
12) Walk in a crowded mall with people walking past you?
13) Get bumped by people as you walk in a mall?
14) Step on or off an escalator while holding onto a railing?

15) Step on or off an escalator while holding parcels & not holding a railing?

16) Walk outside on icy sidewalks?

Now add up your total score (the maximum is 1600) and divide by 16. This will give you an overall balance confidence percentage. The table below indicates your level of balance functionality based on your percentage:

ABC Score	Balance Level
80-100%	Highly functional
50-80%	Moderately functional
0-50%	Low functionality

Key Point Summary:
- Before beginning a balance training program, test your current level of balance.
- Perform the following static tests:
    - Standing Cushion Test
    - Standing Feet Together Test
    - Standing Feet Together Test (eyes closed)
    - Semi Tandem Stance Test
    - Tandem Stance Test
    - Single Leg Test

Single Leg test with Arm Curls
- Perform the following movements tests:

    TUG Test

    5X Sit to Stand Test

    Six Minute Walk Test
- Take the ABC Balance Confidence Scale Test

In the next chapter, we'll lay out a plan for a holistic exercise program to cover all aspects of fitness.

* * *

Chapter Four:

Let's Make a Plan

"Even if you're on the right track, you'll get run over if you just sit there!"

Will Rogers

A Holistic Approach to Senior Fitness

There are very few things that most people agree on nowadays. Things we considered no-brainer facts just a generation ago are now being questioned. But there is one statement we can't argue with - the evidence to support it is just too overwhelming.

Here it is …

The fitter you are in old age, the more healthy, mobile, and balanced you will be.

As a personal fitness trainer, it is gratifying to see many elderly people embracing fitness. More and more elderly folks are joining gyms, playing sports like pickleball and walking soccer, and taking up walking as an exercise habit.

But there is something else that I have noticed. Many people, across all generations, tend to focus on one or two elements of fitness and neglect the others. That is not the way to develop total fitness - and total fitness should be your goal regardless of age.

Even though this book zones in on one specific element of the six pillars of fitness - balance - I want to encourage you to adopt a holistic approach to develop total fitness. That's why, in this chapter, I will briefly lay out a comprehensive fitness program to help you to improve in every area of your life.

There are 6 pillars of total fitness:

1. Strength
2. Flexibility
3. Mobility / Balance
4. Stability
5. Agility
6. Endurance

When you look at that list, you might think 'I can't do half a dozen different types of exercise to cover off each of those things.'

The good news is that you don't have to.

When you choose the right types of exercise and do them the right way, you will be able to include several aspects at one time.

Let's briefly consider each of these pillars, along with recommendations on how to add them to your routine.

Strength

For a long time strength training and seniors haven't really gone together. Lifting weights has been seen as a young man's game. Fortunately, science has caught up with reality and experts agree that strength training is the single most important thing seniors can do to enhance their physical quality of life.

Strength training has been shown to improve each of the following conditions:

- Arthritis
- Poor balance
- Diabetes
- Osteoporosis
- Obesity
- Back pain
- Breathing problems
- Depression
- Dementia

I recommend beginning a strength training program two times per week, with a three day gap between sessions. You can join a gym, in which case I recommend having a few sessions with a certified personal trainer, or if that's not accessible and financially feasible, you can consider home alternatives. Bodyweight, resistance band, and dumbbell workouts are all excellent options that you can try at home.

Flexibility

Flexible muscles, ligaments, and tendons are stretchy and pliable. Lack of flexibility makes everyday tasks more challenging, decreasing your range of motion and increasing your injury risk if you over-stretch the muscle.

Seniors most commonly experience flexibility problems through the hips and spine. The back pain that results may result from inflexibility in the hamstrings, glutes, and hip flexors. Tightness in these areas will pull the torso downward, producing lower back tension.

Tightness in muscles such as the iliopsoas in the inner part of the hip will cause you to compress your spine and tilt your pelvis forward - again leading to tension in the lower back.

The piriformis muscle is situated in the buttocks above the hip joint. It assists the hip flexors in lifting and moves the thighs away from the body. Lack of flexibility can lead to piriformis syndrome, characterized by numbness and pain in the buttocks. As a result of the piriformis muscle pressing down on the sciatic nerve, many people also experience pain running down each leg, known as sciatica.

You don't have to perform a separate workout to improve your flexibility. Strength training will improve your flexibility as you move a muscle through its full range of motion. Adding dynamic stretching exercises into your balance training sessions as part of your warm-up and a few static stretches after your strength workouts will also enhance your flexibility.

We will build targeted stretches into the workout program detailed in chapter 11.

Mobility / Balance

Mobility relates to the distance and direction that your joints move. It goes hand in hand with balance, with mobility being your ability to get up and move in your environment and balance being their ability to control that movement. The exercises in this book are designed to improve both your mobility and your balance.

Stability

Instability happens when some of our muscles are stronger and more flexible than others. This causes some muscles to be overactive and others to be underactive. As we favor our stronger muscles, the imbalance becomes worse and worse. As a result, we become less and less stable.

Stability training focuses on how to stabilize the body and how to move correctly. It prepares a person to react with optimized reflexes to any situation while maintaining proper joint alignment.

There are two aspects to improving your stability:
- Active stability training
- Passive stability training

Active stability is improved with balance exercises, such as those covered in this book.

Passive stability is about the movement of your bones, ligaments, and cartilage. These will be strengthened as a result of your strength training workouts.

So long as you are exercising all of your muscles and training each side of the body equally (dumbbells are recommended for this), you can overcome the muscular instability that most people develop throughout their lives.

Agility

Agility relates to the ability to move freely and easily. An agile person is more likely to be able to correct themselves if they begin to stumble. Training for improved agility involves a change of direction and quick stop and start movements that encourage the body to work together as a complete unit. It also enhances hand-eye coordination to improve reaction time.

The best way to increase your agility is with what is known as plyometric exercise. Otherwise known as jump training or ballistics, plyometrics involves jumping and quick lateral movement.

As a senior, you need to approach plyometrics cautiously. After all, your joints are not what they once were. Start with an evaluation to assess whether you're ready to do some simple plyometric exercises.

 A simple test is to take hold of a resistance band and stretch it overhead. From here, squat down to full knee bend and then raise straight back up.

If you experience any movement limitation or discomfort while making this move, you should continue to improve your mobility before you move into plyometric training.

If you can perform the test without difficulty, I recommend introducing plyometrics in the form of step-ups.

Endurance

When it comes to your muscles, endurance is the ability to exert force over an extended period of time. Cardiovascular endurance allows you to keep going without getting puffed out. When the grandkids come over, you will have the energy to get active with them without feeling out of breath afterwards.

Muscular endurance training, in which you use a lighter load for higher repetitions, will increase the health of your bones and joints. The reduced likelihood of muscular fatigue will also lessen your likelihood of suffering a fatigue related injury or accident.

To improve your muscular and cardiovascular endurance, you should include a range of repetitions on your resistance training sessions, going as high as 50 reps with a weight that is challenging for the past 10 reps. Participating in sports like pickleball, walking soccer and golf will improve your cardio fitness.

Balance Friendly Footwear

The right pair of shoes can help you to feel more stable on your feet. Here are some things to consider when shopping for balance friendly footwear:

- A wide and flat toe box - this allows you to spread out your toes to increase your base of support. You should also avoid shoes that turn up at the toes, forcing the toes to be lifted as you walk.

- Low heel - an elevated heel alters your body's alignment, bringing the hips and pelvis forward toward the toes. That's not good for balance, which is promoted when the weight is back over your heels.

- Sole flexibility - the more freedom of movement the many bones, muscles and joints in your feet have, the better they will be able to do their job of keeping you stable. A suitably flexible shoe should bend and twist in your hands quite easily.

The Elements of a Comprehensive Balance Program

Now that we've identified the six pillars of a holistic fitness program, let's think about how you can construct an exercise schedule to include all of them. As I mentioned earlier, you don't need to do separate workouts for each of the six pillars; they are all related and weave in and out of each other.

Here is what I recommend you do each week:

- 4 x Balance Drills
- 1 x Agility Training
- 4 x Strength Training
- 1 x Cardio Endurance
- 4 x Static Stretching

The following weekly schedule presents a way to include each of these elements in a balanced way that allows for sufficient recovery and recuperation between workouts.

Mon	Tues	Wed	Thurs	Fri	Sat	Sun
Balance Drills	*Balance Drills*	Agility Training	*Balance Drills*	*Balance Drills*	Cardio Endurance	**Rest**
Strength Upper Body	**Strength Lower Body**	Stability Drills	**Strength Upper Body**	**Strength Lower Body**		
Plus: 5 mins Static Stretching	*Plus:* 5 mins Static Stretching		*Plus:* 5 mins Static Stretching	*Plus:* 5 mins Static Stretching		

Key Point Summary:

A comprehensive holistic exercise program needs to include:

- Fitness
- Flexibility
- Balance
- Stability
- Agility
- Endurance

In the next chapter, we'll lay out a five minute warm-up that you should do before every balance training session.

* * *

Chapter Five:

The Warm Up

"For the unlearned, old age is winter; for the learned, it is the season of the harvest."

Hasidic saying

We all know that we should warm up before exercise. Many people, however, ignore the warm-up, eager to get into the 'meat' of their workout. As a younger person, you may be able to get away with that.

But not as a senior.

Even if your workout involves doing exercises sitting in a chair, you must spend a few minutes transitioning your body from a passive to an active state. Warming up will move more blood from your organs to your muscles, making them more effective in the upcoming workout and reducing the risk of injury.

In a sedentary state, about 20 percent of your body's blood is contained in your skeletal muscle tissue. Performing dynamic stretching exercises will increase that to more than 50 percent. This increased blood supply brings oxygen and nutrients into the muscle cells to energize your workout.

At the same time, dynamic stretching will lubricate the joints and move your muscles through their full range of motion to ready them for the work ahead.

Dynamic vs Static Stretching

When most people think of stretching, they have static stretching in mind. This involves holding a stretch position as you feel slight discomfort in the muscle with the goal of increasing the range of motion.

This is the type of stretching that was traditionally done before exercise. In recent years, however, a large body of research has shown that static stretching before exercise is not a good idea. Not only has static stretching been shown not to improve performance or prevent injury, but it will also actually make you weaker and less supple. [10]

Instead of static stretching before you should take a few minutes to do some dynamic stretching. This involves moving a muscle through its full range of motion for between 10 and 15 repetitions. This type of stretching has been shown to decrease muscle and joint stiffness, improve flexibility and range of motion, increase blood flow to the muscles and help prevent injury. [11]

Dynamic stretching is superior because it allows your body to mimic the pattern of movement that you are likely to perform, which makes your nerve system more efficient at executing the movement, coordinating your various muscles to work together, and controlling the range of motion.

On the other hand, static stretching can be unnatural for your body and may result in muscle damage, or it may make your tissues "too flexible." A certain level of stiffness is required of your muscles when you are doing demanding physical exercises. Static stretching is not bad in all cases, but we should be more careful and selective when choosing such exercises to achieve the best possible results.

7 Dynamic Stretches Your Should Do

The following dynamic stretches will provide an ideal warm up for your balance workouts. If you need to use a chair for support while doing the lower body stretches, feel free to do so.

Arm Circles x 20

1. Stand with your arms out at your sides, in line with your shoulders.
2. Rotate from the shoulder joint to move your arms in small circles.
3. Keep the elbows locked and concentrate on achieving a 360 degree range of motion.
4. Change the direction halfway through. Slow down if you feel stiff, and out of mobility at any point during the 360 degree rotation.

Hip Rotation x 5

1. Stand with your feet shoulder width apart. 2
2. Lift one leg into the air and rotate from the hip to perform a hip circle in a clockwise direction.
3. After 5 rotations, reverse the motion to perform 5 anti-clockwise hip rotations.
4. Repeat on the other leg.

Knee Circles x 5

1. Stand with feet shoulder width apart and hands on hips.
2. Lift one foot slightly off the ground and begin to draw a circle in the air with your knee. The movement will be smaller than in the previous stretch.
3. Perform 5 clockwise followed by 5 anti-clockwise circles.
4. Repeat on the other leg.

Ankle Circles x 5

1. Stand with feet shoulder width apart and hands on hips.
2. Lift one foot slightly off the ground and begin to draw circles with your ankles. This will be the smallest circle yet. Make sure to spread out your toes as you are performing your ankle circles.
3. Perform 5 clockwise followed by 5 anti-clockwise circles.

4. Repeat on the other leg.

Shoulder Shrugs x 10

1. Stand with your arms extended out to your sides at shoulder level.

2. Shrug your shoulder blades up and down. This will warm up your shoulder joint and your trapezius muscles. Do this 10 times.

3. Maintaining the same arms extended position, hold up your thumbs and then rotate at the wrist, supinating and pronating the hands up and down. Do not bend at the elbows as you do this. Do this 10 times.

Shoulder Circles x 5

1. Stand in a neutral position with your arms level with your shoulders, extended away from your body.

2. Keeping your shoulders relaxed, make small circles by rotating your arms backwards five times and then forwards 5 times.

Bear Hug x 10

1. Stand with your arms at your sides. Bring them across your body to cross over and then extend them back to stretch out your pectoral muscles.

2. In the extension, arch your back to feel the movement through your latissimus dorsi muscles. This action basically involves hugging yourself. Do this for 10 repetitions.

Give Your Feet Some Love

Your feet are the foundation of your movements. For most of us, though, our feet have taken quite a beating over the years. Constantly wedging them into shoes, walking on artificial terrain, and being immobile for too long can lead to weakened, out-of-shape foot muscles, ligaments, and bones. This can cause a chain reaction of problems leading to your ankles, knees, hips, and all the way to your neck.

The good news is that, with the right exercises performed on a regular basis, you can quickly strengthen your feet. This will, in turn, improve your balance and coordination.

Here are 5 of the best ...

1. Heel Stretch
    - Sit on the front edge of a chair with your feet flat on the floor and upper body upright, with an arched lower back.
    - Come up on your left heel, tucking your toes in.
    - Lower and repeat.
    - Do this 5 times on each foot.
2. Top of the Foot Stretch

- Sit on the front edge of a chair with your feet flat on the floor and upper body upright, with an arched lower back.
- Lift your left heel and rest on the knuckles of the toes with the toes curled back.
- Hold for 3 seconds.
- Do this 5 times on each foot.

3. Ball Massage
   - Sit on the front edge of a chair with your feet flat on the floor and upper body upright, with an arched lower back.
   - Place a tennis ball on the floor under your left foot.
   - Put your weight fully on the ball and begin massaging your soles from left to right and back and forth.Cover ever part of the foot.
   - Massage your left foot for 60 seconds and then switch to the right foot.

4. Toe Stretch
   - The wider your feet, the larger your base of support will be. This exercise is designed to enhance your balance base.
   - Stand in bare feet with your feet shoulder width apart and hands by your sides.

- Now consciously spread the toes of both feet apart as wide as possible and plant them down on the floor.
- Hold the toe spread position for 15 seconds.
- Do this 5 times.

5. Individual Toe Lifts

    - Stand in bare feet with your feet shoulder width apart and hands by your sides.
    - Practice individual toe control by lifting both big toes into the air while keeping all of the other toes down. Hold for a count of 5.
    - Now lift only your right big toe directly up, holding it up for a count of 5.
    - Repeat with the left big toe.
    - Next, bring up the big and second toe, keeping the balls of the feet down. Hold them up for a 5 second count.

We will include these exercises in our weekly program, detailed in Chapter 11.

Key Point Summary:
- Begin every session with a warm-up
- Your balance training exercise warm-up should consist of dynamic stretching exercises.

In the next chapter, we'll lay out 10 super effective exercises to strengthen your core, which is central to improving balance.

* * *

Chapter Six:

Core Balance

"Aging is not lost youth but a new stage of opportunity and strength."

Betty Friedman

Why You Need a Strong Core

The most important part of your spine for balance and stability is the area from the lower lumbar spine to the pelvis. The weight that is transferred down through the spine is being pulled directly down by the force of gravity. However, that weight needs to be transferred laterally to either side of the pelvis. The large pelvic joints that transfer that weight are not stable - in fact, they are very wobbly.

The wobbly, unstable nature of the pelvic joints and the spine presents a challenge in terms of balance when we move. Fortunately, we have a built-in support structure in the form of the core muscles.

That's why a poor posture, and a lack of core strength can often lead to lower back pain, because an immense amount of pressure to keep your body stable is put on that region, without other muscle groups helping with the effort.

The core muscles are the:

- Erector spinae, which runs up and down the length of your spine
- Psoas, which connects to the front of the lower spine and runs down to the hips
- Gluteus muscles of the buttocks
- Rectus abdominis, which is the front wall of your stomach
- External obliques, which passes obliquely down from the ribcage to the pelvic bone
- Internal obliques, which passes obliquely upward from the pelvic bone to the ribs
- Transverse abdominis, which lies horizontally across the abdominal wall

The more solid your core is, the more stable your pelvic bones will be when you stand and move. So, the stronger the muscles that make up your core, the less stress will be placed on the pelvic girdle and the more balanced, mobile, and agile you will be.

The more stable your core is, the more efficiently you can sit, stand, and transition between the two. When you're sitting, the base of your posture is your pelvis. If you allow your pelvis to roll back, you go into a seat curve position. Your back will be rounded, placing less stress on the lower spine. As a result, you will be reducing the likelihood of having to put up with ongoing lower back pain.

By rolling the pelvis forward, your spine will straighten out to assume its neutral s-curve position. This allows you to maintain a slight lumbar curve in the small of your back.

The tighter your abdominal wall, and the stronger your erector spinae, the more naturally you will assume this position in a seated and standing position. This will allow you to move from the hip joint rather than the spine. When you get out of a seated position, you'll be able to get your center of gravity over your base of support while keeping your core stable. At the same time, you should shift your weight forward to use the large muscles in your quadriceps to come up to a standing position.

10 Core Exercises

As you are doing these core exercises, you should be taking deep breaths in through your nose and exhaling through your mouth. Remain nice and tall for each exercise, maintaining a natural low back arch and pulling your shoulders back.

1. **Core Brace**
   1. Sit upright on the edge of a chair with your feet firmly on the floor. Tighten your core by pulling in your lower back and tensing your abdominal muscles. Place your hands on your thighs.
   2. Now pull your belly button in towards your spine.
   3. Hold this tight core position for 10 seconds and then relax for 3 seconds.

4. Do this 10 times.

2. Seated Twist

1. Sit upright on the edge of a chair with your feet firmly on the floor. Tighten your core by pulling in your lower back and tensing your abdominal muscles. Place your hands on your thighs.
2. Now fold your arms and bring them up to shoulder level. Rotate to the left as far as you can. Then return to the center and rotate to the right..
3. Do this 10 times on each side.

3. Seated Butterfly

1. Sit upright on the edge of a chair with your feet firmly on the floor. Tighten your core by pulling in your lower back and tensing your abdominal muscles. Bring your arms up to shoulder level with your elbows bent at a 45 degree angle and your palms facing forward.
2. Now bring your arms together to meet in front of your chest.
3. Squeeze your hands together.
4. Return to the start position. Try to keep your elbows parallel to the floor as you do this exercise.
5. Do this 10 times.

4. Seated Reach

1. Sit upright on the edge of a chair with your feet wide apart. Tighten your core by pulling in your lower back

and tensing your abdominal muscles. Place your hands on your thighs.

2. Now reach your right hand out to the side to stretch the side of your torso. Imagine that you are reaching for a jar that is on the table just beyond your reach.

3. Alternate reaching to the right and left hand side, being sure to maintain an upright torso position throughout.

4. Do this 10 times.

5. Reverse Sit Up

1. Sit upright on the edge of a chair with your knees together and feet out about two feet from the chair. Tighten your core by pulling in your lower back and tensing your abdominal muscles. Cross your hands over your chest.

2. Now, maintaining a natural arch in your lower back, lean back toward the chair back support.

3. Stop just short of touching the chair back and then come back to an upright position, using your core muscles to pull you up.

4. Do this 10 times.

6. Knee Lift Reach

1. Sit upright on the edge of a chair with your knees together and feet out about two feet from the chair. Tighten your core by pulling in your lower back and

tensing your abdominal muscles. Cross your hands over your chest.

2. Lean back to rest your shoulder blades on the chair back. Position your arms out to the sides with your elbows bent.

3. Now lift your left knee up off the floor. At the same time, reach your right hand across the left knee.

4. Alternate from side to side, pulling in your belly button as you reach across.

5. Do this 10 times on each side.

7. Knee Lift

1. Sit upright on the edge of a chair with your knees together and feet out about two feet from the chair. Tighten your core by pulling in your lower back and tensing your abdominal muscles. Imagine that you are leveling your lower back to the ground.

2. Now lean your shoulders back to rest on the chair back support. Grab the sides of the chair seat with your hands.

3. Lift your right knee up as high as you can and then lower in back down.

4. Alternate from side to side, planting your foot firmly back on the floor each time.

5. Do this 10 times on each side.

8. Side Reach

1. Sit upright on the edge of a chair with your knees together and feet out about two feet from the chair. Tighten your core by pulling in your lower back and tensing your abdominal muscles. Place your left hand on your knee and hang your right arm by your side.
2. Reach your right hand down to the floor to stretch the sides of your waist. Keep your shoulders and hips straight and your core tight.
3. Do this 10 times on each side.

9. Heel Toe Taps

1. Sit upright on the edge of a chair with your knees together. Tighten your core by pulling in your lower back and tensing your abdominal muscles. Your feet should be firmly planted on the floor.
2. Bring your feet back under the chair to tap your toes to the floor.
3. Immediately extend your legs to tap your heels to the floor.
4. Do this alternating toe-heel tap movement 10 times.

10. Bicycle

1. Sit upright on the edge of a chair with your knees together and feet out about two feet from the chair. Tighten your core by pulling in your lower back and tensing your abdominal muscles. Hold the sides of the chair seat for support.

2. Maintaining a natural arch in your lower back, lean back toward the chair back support, stopping just short of touching it.

3. Now, imagine that you're riding a bike, bringing your feet off the ground and doing a pedaling motion in the air. Pedal 5 times forward and five times back.

In the next chapter, we move into our dedicated balance program with 12 general purpose and 3 arthritis specific seated balance exercises.

* * *

Chapter Seven:

Phase One: Seated Exercises

"It does not matter how slowly you go as long as you do not stop."

Confucious

The key to an effective exercise program is to begin at a level accessible to you and then gradually and progressively increase the difficulty until it becomes more challenging. Seated exercises are a smart entry point for seniors. They allow you to develop a base of strength and flexibility without putting stress on your joints.

The 12 general-purpose seated exercises that follow are designed for able-bodied seniors as well as those who are recovering from a fall, have had a stroke, or have trouble standing. They are followed by three exercises that are specifically designed for people who suffer from arthritis.

Begin by doing just one set of each exercise. The recommended repetitions and length of holds are your starting point. As you get stronger and feel more confident, you should increase the sets and repetitions to a maximum of 3 sets of 15 repetitions or 25-second holds.

For some of these exercises, you will need a plastic cup.

Before beginning these exercises, run through the dynamic warm-up stretches that we covered in Chapter 5. Here's a reminder of those stretches:

- Arm circles x 5
- Hip rotations x 5
- Knee circles x 5
- Ankle circles x 5
- Shoulder shrugs x 10
- Shoulder circles x 5
- Dynamic swimmer stretch x 10

12 General Purpose Exercises

1. Cup Tap

1. Put a plastic cup on the floor in front of your chair.
2. Sit upright on the edge of the chair with your feet firmly on the floor, so that the cup is between them. Tighten your core by pulling in your lower back and tensing your abdominal muscles. Place your hands on your thighs.
3. Tap your right foot on top of the cup and then bring it down to tap the floor on the other side.
4. Reverse this movement to tap the cup again and return the foot to its starting position.
5. Do this 5 times on each foot.

2. Leg Lift/Hold

1. Sit upright on the edge of a chair with your feet firmly on the floor. Tighten your core by pulling in your lower back and tensing your abdominal muscles. Place your hands on the edges of the chair.
2. Bring your right bent right knee up so that it is parallel with your hip and the foot is a few inches off the floor.
3. Hold this position for a 5 second count.
4. Do this 5 times on each leg.

3. Seated Marching

1. Sit upright on the edge of a chair with your feet firmly on the floor. Tighten your core by pulling in your lower back and tensing your abdominal muscles. Place your hands on the edges of the chair.
2. Bring your right bent right knee up so that it is parallel with your hip and the foot is a few inches off the floor.
3. Lower the right leg and bring the left knee up to produce a seated marching action.
4. Continue for 20 total marches, be sure to maintain an upright torso position throughout.

4. Cup Reach

1. Sit upright on the edge of a chair with your feet firmly on the floor and a plastic cup in your left hand. Tighten your core by pulling in your lower back and tensing your abdominal muscles.

2. Straight your right arm out in front of you and place the cup upside down in the palm of that hand.

3. Focus on the cup as you move your arm out to the side as far as you can. Then bring it back to the start position.

4. Do this 5 times on each arm.

Note: If you have limited shoulder mobility, just go to the point that is comfortable for you.

5. Blind Cup Reach

1. Sit upright on the edge of a chair with your feet firmly on the floor and a plastic cup in your left hand. Tighten your core by pulling in your lower back and tensing your abdominal muscles.

2. Straight your right arm out in front of you and place the cup upside down in the palm of that hand.

3. Now close your eyes!

4. Focus on the cup as you move your arm out to the side as far as you can. Then bring it back to the start position.

5. Do this 5 times on each arm.

6. Seated Arm and Leg Lift

1. Sit upright on the edge of a chair with your feet firmly on the floor. Tighten your core by pulling in your lower back and tensing your abdominal muscles.

2. Lift both your right arm and left foot into the air. Hold for 2 seconds.

3. Lower and repeat with the left arm and right foot.

4. Do this 5 times on each side.

7. Puppet Stretch

1. Sit upright on the edge of a chair with your feet firmly on the floor. Tighten your core by pulling in your lower back and tensing your abdominal muscles.

2. Bring your arms up to shoulder level with elbows bent at 90 degrees. Your arms should be hanging down like a puppet. Allow your elbows to flare out wide.

3. Maintaining an upright body with your shoulder blades pulled back, lowering your arms to full extension, and flexing out your fingers in the bottom position.

4. Draw your elbows back up to the puppet position.

5. Do this 10 times on each side.

8. Rope Climb

1. Sit upright on the edge of a chair with your feet firmly on the floor. Tighten your core by pulling your lower back and tensing your abdominal muscles.

2. Lift both arms above your head, imagining that you are grabbing onto a rope directly above you.

3. Simulate climbing the rope. Bring one hand up as the other elbow goes down. Look up as you climb.

4. Do 10 climbs on each arm, keeping your torso upright throughout.

9. Leg Extensions

1. Sit upright on the edge of a chair with your feet firmly on the floor. Tighten your core by pulling your lower back and tensing your abdominal muscles. Place your hands on your knees.
2. Extend your left leg out in front of you, stopping short of full knee extension. Now draw it back in.
3. Repeat with the right leg.
4. Alternate until you have done 10 leg extensions on each leg.

10. Leg Openers

1. Sit upright on the edge of a chair with your feet firmly on the floor. Tighten your core by pulling in your lower back and tensing your abdominal muscles. Place your hands together in front of your body.
2. Keeping your torso centralized, step your right foot out to the side and then back in. Move the corresponding hand to the side to match your foot movement.
3. Repeat with left foot, alternating 10 times on each leg.

11. Seated In & Outs

1. Sit upright on the edge of a chair with your feet firmly on the floor. Tighten your core by pulling in your lower

back and tensing your abdominal muscles. Bring your elbows into the sides of your body, bent at 90 degrees.

2. Simultaneously bring your arms and feet out to the side. Keep your elbows in at the sides of your body as the hands open apart as far as possible. At the same time open up your feet.
3. Maintaining a tight core, bring your hands and feet back to the center position.
4. Do this 10 times.

12. Calf/Tibia Raises

1. Sit upright on the edge of a chair with your feet shoulder distance apart. Tighten your core by pulling in your lower back and tensing your abdominal muscles. Place your hands on your knees
2. Lift up onto your toes to feel a stretch in the calf muscles. Hold the top position for a second and lower your heel back to the floor.
3. Do this 5 times.
4. Now lift your toes so that you are only resting on your heels. Hold the top position for a second then lower.
5. Do this 5 times.

3 Arthritis Friendly Exercises

1. Hip Abduction

1. Sit upright on the edge of a chair with your feet together. Tighten your core by pulling in your lower back and tensing your abdominal muscles. Place your hands on your knees.
2. Spread your knees apart as far as you comfortably can while keeping the feet together.
3. Do this 10 times.

2. External Rotation

1. Sit upright on the edge of a chair with your feet together. Tighten your core by pulling in your lower back and tensing your abdominal muscles.
2. Cross your right foot over your left knee, so the ankle is resting on the knee. Put your right hand on the right knee.
3. Gently work the knee up and down to externally rotate the hip.
4. Work the knee up and down 10 times and then do the other side.

Note: If you can't cross your leg onto the opposite knee, you can simply work the knee up and down with your foot on the floor.

3. Plantar Flexion

1. Lean back in your chair to rest your shoulder against the back support.
2. Extend your legs out in front of you, resting on your heels.
3. Tap your toes to the floor and then pull them back up as high as you can.
4. Do this 10 times.

In the next chapter, we gradually increase the challenge with 12 general purpose and 3 arthritis specific standing balance exercises.

* * *

Chapter Eight:

Phase Two: Standing Exercises

"Beautiful young people are accidents of nature, but beautiful old people are works of art."

Eleanor Roosevelt

Standing provides an extra element to your workout, making it more challenging. It requires more stability and balance to perform and are more dynamic. This makes them more functional, helping you to be more confident when carrying out everyday tasks.

These exercises will more effectively strengthen your lower body muscles than seated exercises. Feel free to hold onto the back of the chair or other support if you need to.

One each of these exercises, you should breathe in through your nose during the first, or concentric, part of the exercise, and out through your mouth on the second, or eccentric, part. Do not hold your breath at any time when doing these or any other exercises.

The recommended repetition count is a starting point. Build up to doing 3 sets of 20 repetitions on each exercise.

12 General Purpose Exercises

1. Heel Raises

1. Stand behind a chair with your feet shoulder width apart and your hands resting lightly on the top of the chair. Stand up straight with your core tight and your shoulders back.
2. Rise up high onto the balls of your feet as high as you can, maintaining just a slight bend in your knees.
3. Lower back down to the start position. Avoid bouncing, slowly raise your heels back, and forth without relying on momentum.
4. As you become more confident, remove one, then the other hands from the chair.
5. Do 15 repetitions

2. Hamstring Curl

1. Stand behind a chair with your feet shoulder width apart and your hands resting lightly on the top of the chair. Stand up straight with your core tight and your shoulders back.
2. Bend the right knee to bring the heel up behind toward your butt. Come up until the lower leg is parallel with the floor.
3. Slowly return to the floor.
4. Do 10 repetitions on each leg.

3. Side Step

1. Stand upright with your back straight and core tight. Your feet should be shoulder width apart.
2. Take a large step to the left with your outside foot and then bring your other foot across to touch ankle to ankle.
3. Now step to the right with the outside foot, following through again to touch the ankles together.
4. Continue this back and forth lateral movement until you have taken 10 steps in total.

4. Marching in Place

1. Stand behind a chair with your arms supported on the chair back. Stand up tall with shoulders back and core tight.
2. Begin marching in place, bringing your knees as high as you comfortably can.
3. Do 20 marches on each leg.

Note: If you feel comfortable doing this exercise with the aid of a chair for support, you may do so.

5. Side Leg Raise

1. Stand behind a chair with your arms supported on the chair back. Stand up tall with shoulders back and core tight.
2. Bring your left leg directly out to the side as far as is comfortable, moving from the hip.

3. Do this 10 times on each leg.

6. Heel/Toe Rock

1. Stand behind a chair with your feet shoulder width apart and your hands resting lightly on the top of the chair. Stand up straight with your core tight and your shoulders back.
2. Rise up high onto the balls of your feet as high as you can, maintaining just a slight bend in your knees.
3. Lower back down to the start position.
4. Now rise up on your heels to lift your toes to the ceiling.
5. Continue to alternate between toe and heel raises for a total of 10 repetitions.

7. Side-to-Side Weight Transfer

1. Stand upright with your back straight and core tight. Your feet should be slightly wider than shoulder width apart and there should be a slight bend in the knees.
2. Transfer all of your weight onto your right foot and lift your left heel off the floor.
3. Now switch your weight to your left foot as your right heel comes off the floor. Keep your body upright and core tight throughout.
4. Alternate from side to side, doing 10 repetitions in total.

Note: as you become more confident, lift the non weighted foot slightly off the floor.

8. Back-to-Front Transfer

1. Stand upright with your back straight and core tight. Your feet should be shoulder width apart and staggered with the right foot in front and the left behind.
2. Place all of your weight on your front foot and bring the left heel up.
3. Now rock back to place all the weight on your back foot and bring the right toe up off the floor. Keep the core tight and shoulders pulled back.
4. Do 10 repetitions.

Note: as you become more confident, lift the non-weighted foot slightly off the ground.

9. Staggered Calf Raise

1. Stand upright with your back straight and core tight. Your feet should be shoulder width apart and staggered with the right foot in front and the left behind.
2. Raise on both toes to fully stretch your calf muscles.
3. Hold the top stretch position for a second and then lower back to the floor.
4. Each repetition show be slow, without bouncing so you increase the tension on the muscles.

5. Do 15 repetitions.

10. Tightrope Walk

1. Stand upright with your back straight and core tight. Your feet should be shoulder width apart and staggered with the right foot in front and the left behind. This time place your rear toe right up to the front heel, as if you were walking on a tightrope.

2. Bring the rear foot forward to place it directly in front of the other foot, heel to toe.

3. Continue this tight rope walking action for five steps.

4. Turn around and return to the start position.

Note: if you are not confident doing the tightrope walk unsupported touch your hand to a chair and just take two paces forward so your hand can remain on the chair for support.

If you are feeling confident, perform the return steps by walking backwards.

11. Tandem Twist

1. Stand upright with your back straight and core tight. Your feet should be shoulder width apart and staggered with the right foot in front and the left behind. Again, place your rear toe right up to the front heel, as if you were walking on a tightrope.

2. Now clasp your hands together in front of your chest with your elbows slightly bent.

3. Now twist your torso to your left, pulling from your core until your hands are diagonally pointed in that direction.

4. Pull back to the central position.

5. Now twist to the left, again pulling from the core until your hands are pointed diagonally.

12. Airplane

1. Stand upright with your back straight and core tight. Your feet should be shoulder width apart and opposite each other. Place your extended arms out to your sides at shoulder height.

2. Bring your right fingertips up toward the ceiling as your left fingertips go down toward the floor until your right hand is as high as is comfortable. Keep your arms straight throughout.

3. Now lower the right fingertips to the floor and lift your left fingertips toward the ceiling.

4. Continue alternating sides for a total or 10 repetitions.

Note: the closer you move your feet together, the more of a balance challenge this exercise becomes.

3 Arthritis Friendly exercises

1. Mini Squats

1. Stand behind a chair with your feet shoulder width apart. Stand upright with a natural arch in your back

and your shoulders pulled back. Hold the chair lightly with your finger tips for support.

2. Hinge at the hips to descend into a partial squat so that your thighs are at a 30 degree angle.

3. Hold this position for 30 seconds, looking directly ahead and tensing your thigh muscles. Do not round your back in the mini squat position.

4. As you become more comfortable in this position, you can remove your hands from the chair.

5. To make the exercise more challenging combine the mini squat with alternating punches. Just be sure to keep your back arched.

2. Tandem Standing

1. Stand behind a chair in an upright position, with your back straight and core tight. Your feet should be staggered with the right foot in front and the left behind. Place your rear toe right up to the front heel, as if you were walking on a tightrope. Hold the chair lightly for support with your finger tips.

2. Hold this tandem position for 30 seconds, simultaneously repeatedly lifting your right arm into the air as high as you can and then back down to your side.

3. Repeat for another 30 seconds, lifting the left arm into the air and back down.

4. As you feel comfortable with this exercise, remove both hands from the chair and bring them up and down together.

3. Tandem Jacks

1. Stand in an upright position, with your back straight and core tight. Your feet should be shoulder width apart and staggered with the right foot in front and the left behind. Place your rear toe right up to the front heel, as if you were walking on a tightrope. Put your hands at your sides with palms facing forward.
2. Bring both arms up overhead to clap the hands together overhead.
3. Lower to the start position and repeat.

In the next chapter, we focus on the vestibular system with a series of exercises designed to improve your sensory processing center functioning.

* * *

Chapter Nine:

Phase Three: Vestibular Exercises

"The best day to start exercising is today. Tomorrow can turn into weeks, months or years."

Mark Dilworth

How the Vestibular System Works

The vestibular system is a sensory processing center that provides the brain with information about motion, head position, and spatial orientation. It also involves motor functions that allow us to keep our balance, stabilize the head and body during movement and maintain our posture.

The key components of the vestibular system are located in the inner ear in a system of compartments known as the vestibular labyrinth. The vestibular labyrinth contains three tubes in the form of semicircular canals. Each of these canals is situated on the plane to which the head can rotate.

Each of the three canals can detect one of the following head movements:

- Nodding up and down
- Shaking side to side

- Tilting left and right

The canals are filled with a fluid called endolymph. When the head is rotated, this causes the movement of endolymph through the canal that corresponds to the plane of movement. The endolymph then flows into an expansion of the canal called the ampulla.

The ampulla contains hair cells. These are the sensory receptors of the vestibular system. At the top of each hair cell is a collection of small hairs called stereocilia. The endolymph's movement causes these stereocilia's movement, which, in turn, leads to the release of neurotransmitters that send information about the plane of movement to the brain.

The vestibular system uses two other organs, known as the otolith organs, to detect forward and backward movements and gravitational forces. There are two otolith organs in the vestibular labyrinth:

- The utricle
- The saccule

The utricle detects movement in the horizontal plane, while the saccule does so in the vertical plane. Within these two organs are hair cells which detect movement when crystals of calcium carbonate called otoconia shift around, leading to movement in the layers below the otoconia and displacement of hair cells.

The Cawthorne-Cooksey Vestibular Balance Exercises

The Cawthorne-Cooksey exercises are a set of exercises that were developed during the Second World War to treat soldiers with balance problems. They are designed to ...

- Train a person's eyes to move independently of the head
- Improve balance in everyday situations
- Relax tense neck and shoulder muscles
- Improve coordination

These exercises target the three main inputs to balance:

- Visual
- Inner ear
- Proprioceptive

The visual system will be targeted to a progression of eye tracking exercises. The inner ear is targeted through exercises that emphasize the vestibulo-ocular reflex. Finally, the proprioception component is targeted through exercises of the neck and the joints in the body.

These exercises are designed to be progressive, so that you advance step-by-step. Safety is paramount when doing these, or any exercises. If at any time you feel unsafe, or feel that you are at risk of falling, stop the exercise immediately.

1. **Eye Tracking**
    1. Sit comfortably in a chair in an upright position.

2. Move your eyes up and down 10 times.
3. Now move your eyes side to side 10 times.
4. Hold a pen in your right hand and focus on it as you bring your hand in to about six inches from your nose and then out 10 times. Repeat with the pen in the left hand.

2. Head Movement

1. Sit comfortably in a chair in an upright position. Hold a pen in your right hand at arm's length and focus on it. While keeping the pen in focus, move your head up and down 10 times.
2. Start slowly, then increase the speed as you become more comfortable.
3. While still focusing on the pen, move your head from side to side. Again start slowly, and then gradually increase the speed.

3. Shoulder Shrug

1. Sit comfortably in a chair in an upright position.
2. Shrug your shoulders backwards and then forwards, alternating between the two.
3. Do 20 total shrugs.

4. Object Pick Up

1. Sit comfortably in a chair in an upright position. Hold an object such as a tennis ball in your right hand.

2. Bend down to the floor to touch the object to the floor. Do not round your back as you come down (maintain a natural arch in your lower back).
3. Come back up to an upright position.
4. Do this 5 times with your right hand and then repeat with your left hand.

The next three exercises are repeats of exercises 1-3, but in a standing position. This introduces an extra element of balance challenge to the movement.

5. Eye Tracking (Standing)

1. Stand tall, pulling your shoulders back and maintaining a natural arch in your spine.
2. Move your eyes up and down 10 times.
3. Now move your eyes side to side 10 times.
4. Hold a pen in your right hand and focus on it as you bring your hand in to about six inches from your nose and then out 10 times. Repeat with the pen in the left hand.

6. Head Movement (Standing)

1. Stand tall, pulling your shoulders back and maintaining a natural arch in your spine.
2. Hold a pen in your right hand at arm's length and focus on it. While keeping the pen in focus, move your head up and down 10 times.

3. Start slowly, then increase the speed as you become more comfortable.

   4. While still focusing on the pen, move your head from side to side. Again start slowly, and then gradually increase the speed.

7. **Shoulder Shrug (Standing)**

   1. Stand tall, pulling your shoulders back and maintaining a natural arch in your spine.

   2. Shrug your shoulders backwards and then forwards, alternating between the two.

   3. Do 20 total shrugs.

8. **Sitting to Standing**

   1. Stand tall in front of a chair, pulling your shoulders back and maintaining a natural arch in your spine. Rest your hands lightly on your thighs.

   2. Sit down in the chair, controlling the descent (don't plonk down).

   3. Stand back up, trying not to push on your thighs with your hands.

   4. Do this 5 times.

9. **Sitting to Standing (Eyes Closed)**

   1. Stand tall in front of a chair, pulling your shoulders back and maintaining a natural arch in your spine. Rest your hands lightly on your thighs. Now close your eyes.

2. Sit down in the chair, controlling the descent (don't plonk down).
3. Stand back up, trying not to push on your thighs with your hands.
4. Do this 5 times.

10. Sitting to Standing with Turn

1. Stand tall in front of a chair, pulling your shoulders back and maintaining a natural arch in your spine. Rest your hands lightly on your thighs. Now close your eyes.
2. Sit down in the chair, controlling the descent (don't plonk down).
3. Stand back up, trying not to push on your thighs with your hands.
4. Now turn around completely before moving into the next sitting/standing repetition.
5. Alternate turning directions each time.
6. 10 ten repetitions in total.
7. Stop if at any time you feel dizzy.

11. Ball Toss

1. Stand tall with a tennis ball in your right hand. Hold both hands at eye level in front of you with elbows bent at 90 degrees, and hands shoulder width apart.
2. Toss the ball across to your left hand.
3. Throw the ball between your two hands.

4. Do this 10 times.

12. Bent Over Ball Toss

   1. Stand tall with a tennis ball in your right hand and your legs staggered. Bend at the waist to bring your torso down to a 30 degree angle. Maintain a natural arch in your spine, without rounding your back
   2. Toss the ball between your legs from your right hand to your left.
   3. Throw the ball between your two hands.
   4. Do this 10 times leading with your right hand then repeat by leading with your left hand.

Make sure that you have a chair, table or other support that you can reach for balance during the following exercises.

13. Standing on One Foot (Eyes Open)

   1. Stand tall, pulling your shoulders back and maintaining a natural arch in your spine. Your arms should be at your sides.
   2. Lift your left foot off the floor by bending your knee.
   3. Hold for 10 seconds.
   4. Do this 3 times.
   5. Repeat with the right foot elevated.

14. Standing on One Foot (Eyes Closed)

   1. Stand tall, pulling your shoulders back and maintaining a natural arch in your spine. Your arms should be at your sides.

2. Now close your eyes.
   3. Lift your left foot off the floor by bending your knee.
   4. Hold for 10 seconds.
   5. Do this 3 times.
   6. Repeat with the right foot elevated.

15. Heel to Toe Walk (Arms Outstretched)

   1. Stand up tall with your feet in a staggered stance, right foot forward. Now place your feet heel to toe.
   2. Lift your arms out to the side, in line with your shoulders.
   3. Begin walking forward in heel to toe fashion.
   4. Walk forward five steps and then turn and return to the start position.

16. Heel to Toe Walk (Eyes Closed)

   1. Stand up tall with your feet in a staggered stance, right foot forward. Now place your feet heel to toe and close your eyes.
   2. Lift your arms out to the side, in line with your shoulders.
   3. Begin walking forward in heel to toe fashion.
   4. Walk forward five steps and then turn and return to the start position.

Walking Balance Exercises

In this section, we progress to more dynamic exercises that combine all three elements of the vestibular system, vision, and proprioception. These exercises are more advanced, so only progress to them if you have mastered the previous progressions and feel confident to try them out.

So far, we have, on the whole, been addressing the elements of balance individually. That's important, but unless they can work together as a seamless whole, you won't completely conquer your balance problems.

Walking adds an extra challenge to your balance and coordination. Every time you take a step, your body has to adjust its equilibrium to the environment.

Make sure that you are maintaining a good posture when you are doing your walking exercises. That means you should be standing upright, with your shoulders pulled back and a natural arch in your lower back. Pull in your tummy to keep your core tight. Look directly ahead, just taking quick glances at the ground as you move forward.

These exercises should be done with another person standing by to assist you. This person should be able-bodied and strong. You should also wear what is called a gait belt. That's a belt that your assistant can easily grab onto to give support without having to grab you by the arm.

The exercises to follow are designed to be done by people who walk unaided or with a cane. If you use a walker, these exercises are not for you.

Obstacle Course

For the next series of exercises you will negotiate your way over an obstacle course. They are designed to help you to remain balanced and confident when you are in public situations like a mall or a crowded room. In these situations, there are lots of distractions to take your attention away from what is in front of you.

The obstacle course should be made up of the following:

- Two long skinny items that you have to step over (such as an umbrella and a walking cane).
- A squishy item you can stand on (such as a cushion).
- A box or platform that you can step onto (it should be 10-12 inches high).

If you have a flight of stairs in your home, you can set up the obstacle course in front of the stairs, top finish at the first step. Place each obstacle about 18 inches apart.

You should have your assistant right alongside as you go through the obstacle course. If necessary, they can hold onto your belt as you walk. You can also use a cane if you need to.

Here is how to go through the obstacle course.

1. Stand before the first obstacle and then begin walking through it, looking down at the obstacles. Take deliberate steps, one at a time.
2. Do not touch the first two obstacles as you move over them.

3. Stand on the third obstacle with both feet.
4. Step up onto the step obstacle with both feet and then turn around.
5. Walk back through the course to the start point.

Progression One

Walk through the obstacle course several times until you feel comfortable. Then start going through it with a more confident stride and without looking down (you should give each obstacle a quick glance).

Progression Two

When you are able to confidently progress through the obstacle course without having to look down at every obstacle, focus your vision on a point directly in front of you, to the left and to the right.

As you go through the obstacle course, shift your vision focus between these three points, only giving the obstacles a brief glance. Imagine that you are making your way through a crowded mall.

Progression Three

The next progression should involve your assistant talking to you as you are going through the obstacle course. The conversation should not be about their balance but a completely different subject. This will provide a real-life distraction, forcing you to multitask by staying in control of your balance while engaging in unrelated conversation.

Progression Four

Once you can confidently go through the course while looking around and engaging in conversation, start going through it in a side-step fashion. We have to do side stepping regularly as we move around our homes and out in public. If we don't train to be able to do it confidently, we are at risk of stumbling.

Stand side on before the first obstacle. Feel free to use a cane, especially if you have had a stroke or a replacement. Take a sideways step to straddle the first obstacle, then follow through with the rear foot to clear the obstacle. Continue taking even sideways steps to complete the course.

If you find that one foot keeps hitting an obstacle, put effort into exaggerating the leg lift to clear it. Pause at the most difficult part of the course and do repeats.

Progression Five

Progression five sees you going through the obstacle course backwards. This is an advanced balance challenge that you should only try when you have confidently progressed through the other four levels. Your assistant should hold onto your gait belt throughout the entire course.

Start at the beginning of the course facing away from it. Look down as you take backward steps through the course. Take your time, stopping as necessary.

When you can confidently walk backwards going through the course, try doing it from the back to the start. Stand on the step, facing away from the course and begin walking back to the beginning.

> Banish the Senior Shuffle
>
> The senior shuffle is that distinctive unsteady walk that is all common among elder people. As I mentioned earlier, rather than making them safer, it is actually contributing to their lack of balance. Overcoming the senior shuffle is largely a confidence thing; the more you do your balance exercises, the less tensed up you will be when you walk.
>
> As you become more confident, you should be freer in your movements. You should then be able to implement the following good walking form cues:
>
> - Keep your feet pointed directly ahead
> - Place your weight back on your heels
> - Untuck your pelvis, to tip the front of it forward
> - Center your ribcage
> - Keep your chin up

7 Walking Exercises

1. Balance Walking

1. Stand with your feet shoulder-width apart and arms out at your sides at shoulder level.

2. Take a step forward with your right leg. As you follow through with your left leg, bring it up in an exaggerated movement. Pausing for a second before bringing it through to the floor.
3. Now take the next step with your right leg, again bringing it through in an exaggerated movement and pushing for a second before following through.
4. Take 20 steps in this manner.

2. Walking Ball Toss

1. Stand with your feet shoulder width apart and a tennis ball in your right hand.
2. Begin walking forward. With each step toss the ball from one hand to the other.
3. Your goal is to walk forward 10 steps without dropping the ball.

3. Walking the Plank

For this exercise, you will need a slightly elevated platform that you can walk on. A length of 2 x 4 inch timber is ideal. Be sure to have your assistant alongside you as you do this exercise. If the constant head turning causes you to start feeling dizzy, you should stop immediately.

1. Stand on the platform in a heel-to-toe staggered stance.
2. Walk to the end of the platform.
3. Turn around and return to the start position.

1. **Dynamic Walking**
   1. Stand with your feet shoulder width apart and arms out at your sides at shoulder level.
   2. Begin walking up and down the length of your living room, gradually turning your head from side to side as you do so. Try not to look down as you walk.
   3. Once you feel confident walking in your home, do this exercise outside. There you will find plenty of things to focus your attention on. Continue the side to side head movement as you walk, focusing on an object for a few seconds and then switching your attention to the other side. Again try not to look down as you walk.

5. **Side Step Walk**
   1. Stand with your feet together, and your hands clasped together at chest level. Maintain an upright posture.
   2. Take a step to the left with the left foot and follow through with the right foot to bring your feet back together. Look in the direction you are moving.
   3. Side step to the left 10 times.
   4. Now reverse direction to side step to the right 10 times to return to the start position.
   5. Once you are feeling confident, begin doing this exercise outside. If you are walking for exercise (I recommend that you do), add some side shuffle walks every few minutes.

6. Heel/Toe Walk

Only do this exercise once your lower body has been warmed up with several minutes of normal walking. This is a challenging exercise, and so you should have your assistant standing close by. Hold on to them or a countertop if you need to. If you feel your calf muscles cramping during this exercise, you should stop and shake your legs out.

1. Stand with your feet together and your hands held at your sides. Maintain an upright posture.
2. Begin walking forward on your heels. Keep your toes flexed up.
3. Take 10 steps forward.
4. Turn around and take 10 steps back, but this time with your heels elevated.

7. Figure 8 / Zigzag Walk

For this exercise, you will have to set up a zigzag to the figure 8 course on the floor. If you have cones, you can use them. If you don't, an object such as a book will suffice. Place six markers at three-foot distances in a left, right zigzag pattern that has you walking at a diagonal of about 30 degrees.

1. Stand with your feet together in front of the first obstacle, with your hands held at your sides. Maintain an upright posture.
2. Start walking through the zigzag course. Try not to look down as you advance.

In the next chapter, we bring all of the exercises together in the form of a complete 16 week balance training program.

* * *

Chapter Ten:

Putting It All Together

"Some people want it to happen, some wish it would happen, others make it happen."

Michael Jordan

Over the previous ten chapters, you have been presented with many balance exercises - 69 of them in total! That has provided you with the tools to dramatically improve your balance, strengthen your core and lower body muscles, and restore your mobility confidence. To achieve those objectives, however, we must take all of those tools and bring them together into a graduated structure you can use.

In this chapter, I will lay out a 16-week program that will provide that graduated structure. You will recall that, in chapter four, I suggested a weekly holistic exercise program that would deliver complete fitness training.

Mon	Tues	Wed	Thurs	Fri	Sat	Sun
Balance Drills	*Balance Drills*	Agility Training	*Balance Drills*	*Balance Drills*	Cardio Endurance	**Rest**
Strength Upper Body	**Strength Lower Body**	Stability Drills	**Strength Upper Body**	**Strength Lower Body**		
Plus: 5 mins Static Stretching	*Plus:* 5 mins Static Stretching		*Plus:* 5 mins Static Stretching	*Plus:* 5 mins Static Stretching		

That program includes balance training four times per week on Monday, Tuesday, Wednesday and Friday. The session times will increase as you add more complex exercises. They will start at around the five minute mark and increase to around 30 minutes in week 16.

Remember to begin each session with a warm-up. Here's a recap of the dynamic stretching exercises you should run through:

- Arm Circles x 20
- Hip Rotation x 5

- Knee Circles x 5
- Ankle Circles x 5
- Shoulder Shrugs x 10
- Shoulder Circles x 5
- Bear Hug x 10

After the warm-up, your balance session will have three distinct parts. The first part is called your Foot Focus, and is designed to strengthen your foot muscles, improve flexibility and widen your base of support.

The second part is your core circuit to develop your core stability, with an emphasis on the abdominals, obliques and erector spinae muscles of the lower back.

Part three will have you progressing through the actual balance exercises.

In each part of the program, consistency and commitment are key. There will be days when you feel worn down, sore from the previous workout, or generally down on motivation.

If that's the case, I want you to close your eyes, and imagine again why you are doing that, whether it's the desire to safely and comfortably have a relaxing walk in the park, play with your grandchildren, or pick up a sport for which you need better coordination and balance. You can also promise yourself that you will only do 1-2 sets of the first two exercises. Usually, once you start, it's much easier to continue.

Inevitably, there will be days when you won't be able to exercise at all for one reason or another. If that's the case, you shouldn't feel like the whole program is ruined. Think of it as a strategic pause, remind yourself that it's not the end of the world, and just pick up where you've left off.

Consistency to many is about showing up every day, and while that'd be the ideal scenario, what matters the most is that over a long time, you show up again and again, even if you pause for some reason.

The holistic and comprehensive program below will work wonderfully with any other strength training, cardio, or sport that you are doing. However, if your priority is improving your balance and reflexes, then make sure you combine them in a way that doesn't compromise your main balance workouts.

16 Week Training Program

Week 1

Monday	Tuesday	Thursday	Friday
Foot Focus: • Heel Stretch - 5X per foot • Top of Foot Stretch - 5X per foot • Ball Massage - 20 secs per foot	Foot Focus: • Toe Stretch - 5X per foot • Individual Toe Lifts - 5X per foot • Ball Massage - 20 secs per foot	Foot Focus: • Heel Stretch - 5X per foot • Top of Foot Stretch - 5X per foot • Ball Massage - 20 secs per foot	Foot Focus: • Toe Stretch - 5X per foot • Individual Toe Lifts - 5X per foot • Ball Massage - 20 secs per foot
Core Circuit: 10X each • Core Brace • Seated Twist • Seated Reach • Reverse Sit Up	Core Circuit: 10X each • Knee Lift Reach • Side Reach • Heel Toe Taps • Bicycle	Core Circuit: 10X each • Core Brace • Seated Twist • Seated Reach • Reverse Sit Up	Core Circuit: 10X each • Knee Lift Reach • Side Reach • Heel Toe Taps • Bicycle

Balance Exercises: 5X each	Balance Exercises: 5X each	Balance Exercises: 5X each	Balance Exercises: 5X each
• Cup Tap • Leg Lift/Hold • Seated Marching • Cup Reach • Blind Cup Reach	• Puppet Stretch • Rope Climb • Leg Extensions • Leg Openers • Seated In & Outs	• Cup Tap • Leg Lift/Hold • Seated Marching • Cup Reach • Blind Cup Reach	• Puppet Stretch • Rope Climb • Leg Extensions • Leg Openers • Seated In & Outs

Week 2

Monday	Tuesday	Thursday	Friday
Foot Focus: • Heel Stretch - 10X per foot • Top of Foot Stretch - 10X per foot • Ball Massage - 30 secs per foot	Foot Focus: • Toe Stretch - 10X per foot • Individual Toe Lifts - 10X per foot • Ball Massage -	Foot Focus: • Heel Stretch - 10X per foot • Top of Foot Stretch - 10X per foot • Ball Massage -	Foot Focus: • Toe Stretch - 10X per foot • Individual Toe Lifts - 10X per foot • Ball Massage - 30 secs per foot

	30 secs per foot	30 secs per foot	
Core Circuit: 10X each • Core Brace • Seated Twist • Seated Reach • Reverse Sit Up	Core Circuit: 10X each • Knee Lift Reach • Side Reach • Heel Toe Taps • Bicycle	Core Circuit: 10X each • Core Brace • Seated Twist • Seated Reach • Reverse Sit Up	Core Circuit: 10X each • Knee Lift Reach • Side Reach • Heel Toe Taps • Bicycle
Balance Exercises: 5X each • Cup Tap • Leg Lift/Hold • Seated Marching • Cup Reach • Blind Cup Reach	Balance Exercises: 5X each • Puppet Stretch • Rope Climb • Leg Extensions • Leg Openers • Seated In & Outs	Balance Exercises: 5X each • Cup Tap • Leg Lift/Hold • Seated Marching • Cup Reach • Blind Cup Reach	Balance Exercises: 5X each • Puppet Stretch • Rope Climb • Leg Extensions • Leg Openers • Seated In & Outs

Week 3

Monday	Tuesday	Thursday	Friday
Foot Focus: • Heel Stretch - 10X per foot • Top of Foot Stretch - 10X per foot • Ball Massage - 40 secs per foot	Foot Focus: • Toe Stretch - 10X per foot • Individual Toe Lifts - 10X per foot • Ball Massage - 40 secs per foot	Foot Focus: • Heel Stretch - 10X per foot • Top of Foot Stretch - 10X per foot • Ball Massage - 40 secs per foot	Foot Focus: • Toe Stretch - 10X per foot • Individual Toe Lifts - 10X per foot • Ball Massage - 40 secs per foot
Core Circuit: 10X each • Core Brace • Seated Twist • Seated Reach • Reverse Sit Up	Core Circuit: 10X each • Knee Lift Reach • Side Reach • Heel Toe Taps • Bicycle	Core Circuit: 10X each • Core Brace • Seated Twist • Seated Reach • Reverse Sit Up	Core Circuit: 10X each • Knee Lift Reach • Side Reach • Heel Toe Taps • Bicycle

Balance Exercises: 10X each	Balance Exercises: 10X each	Balance Exercises: 10X each	Balance Exercises: 10X each
• Cup Tap • Leg Lift/Hold • Seated Marching • Cup Reach • Blind Cup Reach	• Puppet Stretch • Rope Climb • Leg Extensions • Leg Openers • Seated In & Outs	• Cup Tap • Leg Lift/Hold • Seated Marching • Cup Reach • Blind Cup Reach	• Puppet Stretch • Rope Climb • Leg Extensions • Leg Openers • Seated In & Outs

Week 4

Monday	Tuesday	Thursday	Friday
Foot Focus: • Heel Stretch - 15X per foot • Top of Foot Stretch - 15X per foot • Ball Massage - 50 secs per foot	Foot Focus: • Toe Stretch - 15X per foot • Individual Toe Lifts - 15X per foot • Ball Massage -	Foot Focus: • Heel Stretch - 15X per foot • Top of Foot Stretch - 15X per foot	Foot Focus: • Toe Stretch - 15X per foot • Individual Toe Lifts - 15X per foot • Ball Massage -

	50 secs per foot	• Ball Massage - 50 secs per foot	50 secs per foot
Core Circuit: 15X each • Core Brace • Seated Twist • Seated Reach • Reverse Sit Up	Core Circuit:15X each • Knee Lift Reach • Side Reach • Heel Toe Taps • Bicycle	Core Circuit: 15X each • Core Brace • Seated Twist • Seated Reach • Reverse Sit Up	Core Circuit:15X each • Knee Lift Reach • Side Reach • Heel Toe Taps • Bicycle
Balance Exercises: 15X each • Cup Tap • Leg Lift/Hold • Seated Marching • Cup Reach • Blind Cup Reach	Balance Exercises: 15X each • Puppet Stretch • Rope Climb • Leg Extensions • Leg Openers • Seated In & Outs	Balance Exercises: 15X each • Cup Tap • Leg Lift/Hold • Seated Marching • Cup Reach • Blind Cup Reach	Balance Exercises: 15X each • Puppet Stretch • Rope Climb • Leg Extensions • Leg Openers • Seated In & Outs

Week 5

Monday	Tuesday	Thursday	Friday
Foot Focus: • Heel Stretch - 15X per foot • Top of Foot Stretch - 15X per foot • Ball Massage - 60 secs per foot	Foot Focus: • Toe Stretch - 15X per foot • Individual Toe Lifts - 15X per foot • Ball Massage - 60 secs per foot	Foot Focus: • Heel Stretch - 15X per foot • Top of Foot Stretch - 15X per foot • Ball Massage - 60 secs per foot	Foot Focus: • Toe Stretch - 15X per foot • Individual Toe Lifts - 15X per foot • Ball Massage - 60 secs per foot
Core Circuit: 15X each • Core Brace • Seated Twist • Seated Reach • Reverse Sit Up	Core Circuit: 15X each • Knee Lift Reach • Side Reach • Heel Toe Taps • Bicycle	Core Circuit: 15X each • Core Brace • Seated Twist • Seated Reach • Reverse Sit Up	Core Circuit: 15X each • Knee Lift Reach • Side Reach • Heel Toe Taps • Bicycle

Balance Exercises: 10X each	Balance Exercises: 10X each	Balance Exercises: 10X each	Balance Exercises: 10X each
• Calf/Tibia Raise • Heel Raise • Hamstring Curl • Side Step • Marching in Place • Side Leg Raise • Tandem Twist	• Heel Toe Rock • Side to Side Weight Transfer • Back to Front Transfer • Staggered Calf Raises • Tightrope Walk • Airplane	• Calf/Tibia Raise • Heel Raise • Hamstring Curl • Side Step • Marching in Place • Side Leg Raise • Tandem Twist	• Heel Toe Rock • Side to Side Weight Transfer • Back to Front Transfer • Staggered Calf Raises • Tightrope Walk • Airplane

Week 6

Monday	Tuesday	Thursday	Friday
Foot Focus: • Heel Stretch - 15X per foot • Top of Foot Stretch - 15X per foot	Foot Focus: • Toe Stretch - 15X per foot	Foot Focus: • Heel Stretch - 15X per foot	Foot Focus: • Toe Stretch - 15X per foot

• Ball Massage - 60 secs per foot	• Individual Toe Lifts - 15X per foot • Ball Massage - 60 secs per foot	• Top of Foot Stretch - 15X per foot • Ball Massage - 60 secs per foot	• Individual Toe Lifts - 15X per foot • Ball Massage - 60 secs per foot
Core Circuit: 15X each • Core Brace • Seated Twist • Seated Reach • Reverse Sit Up	Core Circuit: 15X each • Knee Lift Reach • Side Reach • Heel Toe Taps • Bicycle	Core Circuit: 15X each • Core Brace • Seated Twist • Seated Reach • Reverse Sit Up	Core Circuit: 15X each • Knee Lift Reach • Side Reach • Heel Toe Taps • Bicycle
Balance Exercises: 10X each • Calf/Tibia Raise • Heel Raise • Hamstring Curl • Side Step	Balance Exercises: 10X each • Heel Toe Rock • Side to Side Weight Transfer	Balance Exercises: 10X each • Calf/Tibia Raise • Heel Raise • Hamstring Curl • Side Step	Balance Exercises: 10X each • Heel Toe Rock • Side to Side Weight Transfer

- Marching in Place
- Side Leg Raise
- Tandem Twist

- Back to Front Transfer
- Staggered Calf Raises
- Tightrope Walk
- Airplane

- Marching in Place
- Side Leg Raise
- Tandem Twist

- Back to Front Transfer
- Staggered Calf Raises
- Tightrope Walk
- Airplane

Week 7

Monday	Tuesday	Thursday	Friday
Foot Focus: • Heel Stretch - 20X per foot • Top of Foot Stretch - 20X per foot • Ball Massage - 60 secs per foot	Foot Focus: • Toe Stretch - 20X per foot • Individual Toe Lifts - 20X per foot • Ball Massage - 60 secs per foot	Foot Focus: • Heel Stretch - 20X per foot • Top of Foot Stretch - 20X per foot • Ball Massage - 60 secs per foot	Foot Focus: • Toe Stretch - 20X per foot • Individual Toe Lifts - 20X per foot • Ball Massage - 60 secs per foot

Core Circuit: 15X each	Core Circuit: 15X each	Core Circuit: 15X each	Core Circuit: 15X each
- Core Brace - Seated Twist - Seated Reach - Reverse Sit Up	- Knee Lift Reach - Side Reach - Heel Toe Taps - Bicycle	- Core Brace - Seated Twist - Seated Reach - Reverse Sit Up	- Knee Lift Reach - Side Reach - Heel Toe Taps - Bicycle
Balance Exercises: 10X each	Balance Exercises: 10X each	Balance Exercises: 10X each	Balance Exercises: 10X each
- Calf/Tibia Raise - Heel Raise - Hamstring Curl - Side Step - Marching in Place - Side Leg Raise - Tandem Twist	- Heel Toe Rock - Side to Side Weight Transfer - Back to Front Transfer - Staggered Calf Raises - Tightrope Walk - Airplane	- Calf/Tibia Raise - Heel Raise - Hamstring Curl - Side Step - Marching in Place - Side Leg Raise - Tandem Twist	- Heel Toe Rock - Side to Side Weight Transfer - Back to Front Transfer - Staggered Calf Raises - Tightrope Walk - Airplane

Week 8

Monday	Tuesday	Thursday	Friday
Foot Focus: • Heel Stretch - 15X per foot • Top of Foot Stretch - 15X per foot • Ball Massage - 60 secs per foot	Foot Focus: • Toe Stretch - 15X per foot • Individual Toe Lifts - 15X per foot • Ball Massage - 60 secs per foot	Foot Focus: • Heel Stretch - 15X per foot • Top of Foot Stretch - 15X per foot • Ball Massage - 60 secs per foot	Foot Focus: • Toe Stretch - 15X per foot • Individual Toe Lifts - 15X per foot • Ball Massage - 60 secs per foot
Core Circuit: 15X each • Core Brace • Seated Twist • Seated Reach • Reverse Sit Up	Core Circuit:15X each • Knee Lift Reach • Side Reach • Heel Toe Taps • Bicycle	Core Circuit: 15X each • Core Brace • Seated Twist • Seated Reach • Reverse Sit Up	Core Circuit:15X each • Knee Lift Reach • Side Reach • Heel Toe Taps • Bicycle

Balance Exercises: 10X each	Balance Exercises: 10X each	Balance Exercises: 10X each	Balance Exercises: 10X each
• Calf/Tibia Raise • Heel Raise • Hamstring Curl • Side Step • Marching in Place • Side Leg Raise • Tandem Twist	• Heel Toe Rock • Side to Side Weight Transfer • Back to Front Transfer • Staggered Calf Raises • Tightrope Walk • Airplane	• Calf/Tibia Raise • Heel Raise • Hamstring Curl • Side Step • Marching in Place • Side Leg Raise • Tandem Twist	• Heel Toe Rock • Side to Side Weight Transfer • Back to Front Transfer • Staggered Calf Raises • Tightrope Walk • Airplane

Week 9

Monday	Tuesday	Thursday	Friday
Foot Focus: • Heel Stretch - 20X per foot • Top of Foot	Foot Focus: • Toe Stretch - 20X per foot • Individual Toe Lifts - 20X per foot	Foot Focus: • Heel Stretch - 20X per foot • Top of Foot	Foot Focus: • Toe Stretch - 20X per foot • Individual Toe Lifts - 20X per foot

Stretch - 20X per foot • Ball Massage - 60 secs per foot	• Ball Massage - 60 secs per foot	Stretch - 20X per foot • Ball Massage - 60 secs per foot	• Ball Massage - 60 secs per foot
Core Circuit: 20X each • Core Brace • Seated Twist • Seated Reach • Reverse Sit Up	Core Circuit: 20X each • Knee Lift Reach • Side Reach • Heel Toe Taps • Bicycle	Core Circuit: 20X each • Core Brace • Seated Twist • Seated Reach • Reverse Sit Up	Core Circuit: 20X each • Knee Lift Reach • Side Reach • Heel Toe Taps • Bicycle
Balance Exercises: 10X each • Eye Tracking • Head Movement	Balance Exercises: 10X each • Sitting to Standing with Turn • Ball Toss • Bent Over Ball Toss	Balance Exercises: 10X each • Eye Tracking • Head Movement	Balance Exercises: 10X each • Sitting to Standing with Turn • Ball Toss • Bent Over Ball Toss

- Shoulder Shrug
- Object Pickup
- Eye Tracking (Standing)
- Head Movement (Standing)
- Shoulder Shrug (Standing)
- Sitting to Standing
- Sitting to Standing (Eyes Closed)

- Standing on One Foot
- Heel to Toe Walk (Arms Outstretched)
- Heel to Toe Walk (Eyes Closed)

- Shoulder Shrug
- Object Pickup
- Eye Tracking (Standing)
- Head Movement (Standing)
- Shoulder Shrug (Standing)
- Sitting to Standing
- Sitting to Standing (Eyes Closed)

- Standing on One Foot
- Heel to Toe Walk (Arms Outstretched)
- Heel to Toe Walk (Eyes Closed)

Week 10

Monday	Tuesday	Thursday	Friday
Foot Focus: • Heel Stretch - 20X per foot • Top of Foot Stretch - 20X per foot • Ball Massage - 60 secs per foot	Foot Focus: • Toe Stretch - 20X per foot • Individual Toe Lifts - 20X per foot • Ball Massage - 60 secs per foot	Foot Focus: • Heel Stretch - 20X per foot • Top of Foot Stretch - 20X per foot • Ball Massage - 60 secs per foot	Foot Focus: • Toe Stretch - 20X per foot • Individual Toe Lifts - 20X per foot • Ball Massage - 60 secs per foot
Core Circuit: 20X each • Core Brace • Seated Twist • Seated Reach • Reverse Sit Up	Core Circuit: 20X each • Knee Lift Reach • Side Reach • Heel Toe Taps • Bicycle	Core Circuit: 20X each • Core Brace • Seated Twist • Seated Reach • Reverse Sit Up	Core Circuit: 20X each • Knee Lift Reach • Side Reach • Heel Toe Taps • Bicycle

Balance Exercises: 10X each	Balance Exercises: 10X each	Balance Exercises: 10X each	Balance Exercises: 10X each
<ul><li>Eye Tracking</li><li>Head Movement</li><li>Shoulder Shrug</li><li>Object Pickup</li><li>Eye Tracking (Standing)</li><li>Head Movement (Standing)</li><li>Shoulder Shrug (Standing)</li><li>Sitting to Standing</li><li>Sitting to Standing</li></ul>	<ul><li>Sitting to Standing with Turn</li><li>Ball Toss</li><li>Bent Over Ball Toss</li><li>Standing on One Foot</li><li>Heel to Toe Walk (Arms Outstretched)</li><li>Heel to Toe Walk (Eyes Closed)</li></ul>	<ul><li>Eye Tracking</li><li>Head Movement</li><li>Shoulder Shrug</li><li>Object Pickup</li><li>Eye Tracking (Standing)</li><li>Head Movement (Standing)</li><li>Shoulder Shrug (Standing)</li><li>Sitting to Standing</li><li>Sitting to Standing</li></ul>	<ul><li>Sitting to Standing with Turn</li><li>Ball Toss</li><li>Bent Over Ball Toss</li><li>Standing on One Foot</li><li>Heel to Toe Walk (Arms Outstretched)</li><li>Heel to Toe Walk (Eyes Closed)</li></ul>

| | (Eyes Closed) | | (Eyes Closed) | |

Week 11

Monday	Tuesday	Thursday	Friday
Foot Focus: • Heel Stretch - 20X per foot • Top of Foot Stretch - 20X per foot • Ball Massage - 60 secs per foot	Foot Focus: • Toe Stretch - 20X per foot • Individual Toe Lifts - 20X per foot • Ball Massage - 60 secs per foot	Foot Focus: • Heel Stretch - 20X per foot • Top of Foot Stretch - 20X per foot • Ball Massage - 60 secs per foot	Foot Focus: • Toe Stretch - 20X per foot • Individual Toe Lifts - 20X per foot • Ball Massage - 60 secs per foot
Core Circuit: 20X each • Core Brace • Seated Twist • Seated Reach	Core Circuit: 20X each • Knee Lift Reach • Side Reach • Heel Toe Taps	Core Circuit: 20X each • Core Brace • Seated Twist • Seated Reach	Core Circuit: 20X each • Knee Lift Reach • Side Reach • Heel Toe Taps

- Reverse Sit Up	- Bicycle	- Reverse Sit Up	- Bicycle
Balance Exercises: 10X each - Obstacle Course - Progression 1 - Balance Walking - Walking Ball Toss - Dynamic Walking - Side Step Walk - Heel/Toe Walk - Zig Zag Walk	Balance Exercises: 20X each - Sitting to Standing with Turn - Ball Toss - Bent Over Ball Toss - Standing on One Foot - Heel to Toe Walk (Arms Outstretched) - Heel to Toe Walk (Eyes Closed)	Balance Exercises: 10X each - Obstacle Course - Progression 1 - Balance Walking - Walking Ball Toss - Dynamic Walking - Side Step Walk - Heel/Toe Walk - Zig Zag Walk	Balance Exercises: 20X each - Sitting to Standing with Turn - Ball Toss - Bent Over Ball Toss - Standing on One Foot - Heel to Toe Walk (Arms Outstretched) - Heel to Toe Walk (Eyes Closed)

Week 12

Monday	Tuesday	Thursday	Friday
Foot Focus: • Heel Stretch - 20X per foot • Top of Foot Stretch - 20X per foot • Ball Massage - 60 secs per foot	Foot Focus: • Toe Stretch - 20X per foot • Individual Toe Lifts - 20X per foot • Ball Massage - 60 secs per foot	Foot Focus: • Heel Stretch - 20X per foot • Top of Foot Stretch - 20X per foot • Ball Massage - 60 secs per foot	Foot Focus: • Toe Stretch - 20X per foot • Individual Toe Lifts - 20X per foot • Ball Massage - 60 secs per foot
Core Circuit: 20X each • Core Brace • Seated Twist • Seated Reach • Reverse Sit Up	Core Circuit: 20X each • Knee Lift Reach • Side Reach • Heel Toe Taps • Bicycle	Core Circuit: 20X each • Core Brace • Seated Twist • Seated Reach • Reverse Sit Up	Core Circuit: 20X each • Knee Lift Reach • Side Reach • Heel Toe Taps • Bicycle

Balance Exercises: 10X each	Balance Exercises: 20X each	Balance Exercises: 10X each	Balance Exercises: 20X each
<ul><li>Obstacle Course - Progression 2</li><li>Balance Walking</li><li>Walking Ball Toss</li><li>Dynamic Walking</li><li>Side Step Walk</li><li>Heel/Toe Walk</li><li>Zig Zag Walk</li></ul>	<ul><li>Sitting to Standing with Turn</li><li>Ball Toss</li><li>Bent Over Ball Toss</li><li>Standing on One Foot</li><li>Heel to Toe Walk (Arms Outstretched)</li><li>Heel to Toe Walk (Eyes Closed)</li></ul>	<ul><li>Obstacle Course - Progression 2</li><li>Balance Walking</li><li>Walking Ball Toss</li><li>Dynamic Walking</li><li>Side Step Walk</li><li>Heel/Toe Walk</li><li>Zig Zag Walk</li></ul>	<ul><li>Sitting to Standing with Turn</li><li>Ball Toss</li><li>Bent Over Ball Toss</li><li>Standing on One Foot</li><li>Heel to Toe Walk (Arms Outstretched)</li><li>Heel to Toe Walk (Eyes Closed)</li></ul>

Week 13

Monday	Tuesday	Thursday	Friday
Foot Focus: • Heel Stretch - 20X per foot • Top of Foot Stretch - 20X per foot • Ball Massage - 60 secs per foot	Foot Focus: • Toe Stretch - 20X per foot • Individual Toe Lifts - 20X per foot • Ball Massage - 60 secs per foot	Foot Focus: • Heel Stretch - 20X per foot • Top of Foot Stretch - 20X per foot • Ball Massage - 60 secs per foot	Foot Focus: • Toe Stretch - 20X per foot • Individual Toe Lifts - 20X per foot • Ball Massage - 60 secs per foot
Core Circuit: 20X each • Core Brace • Seated Twist • Seated Reach • Reverse Sit Up	Core Circuit: 20X each • Knee Lift Reach • Side Reach • Heel Toe Taps • Bicycle	Core Circuit: 20X each • Core Brace • Seated Twist • Seated Reach • Reverse Sit Up	Core Circuit: 20X each • Knee Lift Reach • Side Reach • Heel Toe Taps • Bicycle

Balance Exercises: 10X each	Balance Exercises: 20X each	Balance Exercises: 10X each	Balance Exercises: 20X each
<ul><li>Obstacle Course - Progression 3</li><li>Balance Walking</li><li>Walking Ball Toss</li><li>Dynamic Walking</li><li>Side Step Walk</li><li>Heel/Toe Walk</li><li>Zig Zag Walk</li></ul>	<ul><li>Sitting to Standing with Turn</li><li>Ball Toss</li><li>Bent Over Ball Toss</li><li>Standing on One Foot</li><li>Heel to Toe Walk (Arms Outstretched)</li><li>Heel to Toe Walk (Eyes Closed)</li></ul>	<ul><li>Obstacle Course - Progression 3</li><li>Balance Walking</li><li>Walking Ball Toss</li><li>Dynamic Walking</li><li>Side Step Walk</li><li>Heel/Toe Walk</li><li>Zig Zag Walk</li></ul>	<ul><li>Sitting to Standing with Turn</li><li>Ball Toss</li><li>Bent Over Ball Toss</li><li>Standing on One Foot</li><li>Heel to Toe Walk (Arms Outstretched)</li><li>Heel to Toe Walk (Eyes Closed)</li></ul>

Week 14

Monday	Tuesday	Thursday	Friday
Foot Focus: • Heel Stretch - 20X per foot • Top of Foot Stretch - 20X per foot • Ball Massage - 60 secs per foot	Foot Focus: • Toe Stretch - 20X per foot • Individual Toe Lifts - 20X per foot • Ball Massage - 60 secs per foot	Foot Focus: • Heel Stretch - 20X per foot • Top of Foot Stretch - 20X per foot • Ball Massage - 60 secs per foot	Foot Focus: • Toe Stretch - 20X per foot • Individual Toe Lifts - 20X per foot • Ball Massage - 60 secs per foot
Core Circuit: 20X each • Core Brace • Seated Twist • Seated Reach • Reverse Sit Up	Core Circuit: 20X each • Knee Lift Reach • Side Reach • Heel Toe Taps • Bicycle	Core Circuit: 20X each • Core Brace • Seated Twist • Seated Reach • Reverse Sit Up	Core Circuit: 20X each • Knee Lift Reach • Side Reach • Heel Toe Taps • Bicycle

Balance Exercises: 10X each	Balance Exercises: 20X each	Balance Exercises: 10X each	Balance Exercises: 20X each
- Obstacle Course - Progression 4 - Balance Walking - Walking Ball Toss - Dynamic Walking - Side Step Walk - Heel/Toe Walk - Zig Zag Walk	- Sitting to Standing with Turn - Ball Toss - Bent Over Ball Toss - Standing on One Foot - Heel to Toe Walk (Arms Outstretched) - Heel to Toe Walk (Eyes Closed)	- Obstacle Course - Progression 4 - Balance Walking - Walking Ball Toss - Dynamic Walking - Side Step Walk - Heel/Toe Walk - Zig Zag Walk	- Sitting to Standing with Turn - Ball Toss - Bent Over Ball Toss - Standing on One Foot - Heel to Toe Walk (Arms Outstretched) - Heel to Toe Walk (Eyes Closed)

Week 15

Monday	Tuesday	Thursday	Friday
Foot Focus: - Heel Stretch - 20X per foot	Foot Focus: - Toe Stretch - 20X per foot	Foot Focus: - Heel Stretch - 20X per foot	Foot Focus: - Toe Stretch - 20X per foot

• Top of Foot Stretch - 20X per foot • Ball Massage - 60 secs per foot	• Individual Toe Lifts - 20X per foot • Ball Massage - 60 secs per foot	• Top of Foot Stretch - 20X per foot • Ball Massage - 60 secs per foot	• Individual Toe Lifts - 20X per foot • Ball Massage - 60 secs per foot
Core Circuit: 20X each • Core Brace • Seated Twist • Seated Reach • Reverse Sit Up	Core Circuit: 20X each • Knee Lift Reach • Side Reach • Heel Toe Taps • Bicycle	Core Circuit: 20X each • Core Brace • Seated Twist • Seated Reach • Reverse Sit Up	Core Circuit: 20X each • Knee Lift Reach • Side Reach • Heel Toe Taps • Bicycle
Balance Exercises: 10X each • Obstacle Course - Progression 5 • Balance Walking	Balance Exercises: 20X each • Sitting to Standing with Turn • Ball Toss	Balance Exercises: 10X each • Obstacle Course - Progression 5 • Balance Walking	Balance Exercises: 20X each • Sitting to Standing with Turn • Ball Toss

• Walking Ball Toss • Dynamic Walking • Side Step Walk • Heel/Toe Walk • Zig Zag Walk	• Bent Over Ball Toss • Standing on One Foot • Heel to Toe Walk (Arms Outstretched) • Heel to Toe Walk (Eyes Closed)	• Walking Ball Toss • Dynamic Walking • Side Step Walk • Heel/Toe Walk • Zig Zag Walk	• Bent Over Ball Toss • Standing on One Foot • Heel to Toe Walk (Arms Outstretched) • Heel to Toe Walk (Eyes Closed)

Week 16

Monday	Tuesday	Thursday	Friday
Foot Focus: • Heel Stretch - 20X per foot • Top of Foot Stretch - 20X per foot • Ball Massage - 60 secs per foot	Foot Focus: • Toe Stretch - 20X per foot • Individual Toe Lifts - 20X per foot • Ball Massage - 60 secs per foot	Foot Focus: • Heel Stretch - 20X per foot • Top of Foot Stretch - 20X per foot • Ball Massage - 60 secs per foot	Foot Focus: • Toe Stretch - 20X per foot • Individual Toe Lifts - 20X per foot • Ball Massage - 60 secs per foot

Core Circuit: 20X each • Core Brace • Seated Twist • Seated Reach • Reverse Sit Up	Core Circuit: 20X each • Knee Lift Reach • Side Reach • Heel Toe Taps • Bicycle	Core Circuit: 20X each • Core Brace • Seated Twist • Seated Reach • Reverse Sit Up	Core Circuit: 20X each • Knee Lift Reach • Side Reach • Heel Toe Taps • Bicycle
Balance Exercises: 10X each • Obstacle Course - Progression 5 • Balance Walking • Walking Ball Toss • Dynamic Walking • Side Step Walk • Heel/Toe Walk	Balance Exercises: 20X each • Sitting to Standing with Turn • Ball Toss • Bent Over Ball Toss • Standing on One Foot • Heel to Toe Walk (Arms Outstretched)	Balance Exercises: 10X each • Obstacle Course - Progression 5 • Balance Walking • Walking Ball Toss • Dynamic Walking • Side Step Walk • Heel/Toe Walk	Balance Exercises: 20X each • Sitting to Standing with Turn • Ball Toss • Bent Over Ball Toss • Standing on One Foot • Heel to Toe Walk (Arms Outstretched)

- Zig Zag Walk
- Heel to Toe Walk (Eyes Closed)
- Zig Zag Walk
- Heel to Toe Walk (Eyes Closed)

Conclusion

"Motivation is what gets you started. Habit is what keeps you going."

Jim Ryun

Congratulations. You now have all the tools to reclaim your balance, strengthen your core and lower body muscles and become more confident on your feet. In this book, I have laid out the exercises and training programs I've been using for decades to help seniors regain the balance they thought they had lost forever.

So, you've got the tools. The question is, what are you going to do with them? Statistics tell us that 78 percent of people who buy exercise guides like this one end up absorbing the information but don't achieve long-term results, despite vastly improving their exercise understanding.

Some feel overwhelmed and don't start any of the exercises. Others feel a few sparks of motivation and take action, but with not much progress and dwindling desire to continue, eventually, they stop trying. No matter the individual story, the unfortunate reality is that many people have an intense desire to be better and have all the necessary tools but struggle to take the necessary actions.

The information in this book, along with your need to reclaim your balance - and your confidence - are too important to be left as words on a page. So, here's the question I'd like to leave you with ...

Are you going to be like the 78% of readers of exercise guides and fail to implement what you've learned? Or are you going to break free from the shackles of your mobility issues and take matters into your own hands?

Life is about trying, even in the face of adversity and when you feel as if you won't succeed. I'm not saying that this program will be a magical solution, nor that you should stick with it for the rest of your life. But before you abandon any effort, I encourage you to be a statistical exception and try it out for the full 16 weeks. What you do after that is up to you.

The choice is yours.

Yours in Good Health,

* * *

References

[1] https://www.cdc.gov/steadi/patient.html

[2] Friedman SM, Munoz B, West SK, Rubin GS, Fried LP. Falls and fear of falling: which comes first? A longitudinal prediction model suggests strategies for primary and secondary prevention. J Am Geriatr Soc. 2002 Aug;50(8):1329-35. doi:10.1046/j.1532-5415.2002.50352.x.PMID: 12164987.

[3] Herman T, Giladi N, Gurevich T, Hausdorff JM. Gait instability and fractal dynamics of older adults with a "cautious" gait: why do certain older adults walk fearfully? Gait Posture. 2005 Feb;21(2):178-85. doi: 10.1016/j.gaitpost.2004.01.014. PMID: 15639397.

[4] Liu, C., & Latham, N. K. (2009). Progressive resistance strength training for improving physical function in older adults. The Cochrane Database of Systematic Reviews, (3), CD002759. http://doi.org/10.1002/14651858.CD002759.pub2

[5] Jette AM, Lachman M, Giorgetti MM, Assmann SF, Harris BA, Levenson C, Wernick M, Krebs D. Exercise--it's never too late: the strong-for-life program. Am J Public Health.

1999 Jan;89(1):66-72. doi: 10.2105/ajph.89.1.66. PMID: 9987467; PMCID: PMC1508501.

[6] American College of Sports Medicine (ACSM) (2009b). Exercise and physical activity for older adults. Position stand.Medicine and Science in Sport and Exercise, 41, 1510-1530.

[7] Turner MN, Hernandez DO, Cade W, Emerson CP, Reynolds JM, Best TM. The Role of Resistance Training Dosing on Pain and Physical Function in Individuals With Knee Osteoarthritis: A Systematic Review. Sports Health. 2020 Mar/Apr;12(2):200-206. doi: 10.1177/1941738119887183. Epub 2019 Dec 18. PMID: 31850826; PMCID: PMC7040944.

[8] Enright PL. The six-minute walk test. Respir Care. 2003 Aug;48(8):783-5. PMID: 12890299.

[9] Powell LE, Myers AM. The Activities-specific Balance Confidence (ABC) Scale. J Gerontol A Biol Sci Med Sci. 1995 Jan;50A(1):M28-34. doi: 10.1093/gerona/50a.1.m28. PMID: 7814786.

[10] Simic L, Sarabon N, Markovic G. Does pre-exercise static stretching inhibit maximal muscular performance? A meta-analytical review. Scand J Med Sci Sports. 2013 Mar;23(2):131-48. Doi: 10.1111/j.1600-0838.2012.01444.x. Epub 2012 Feb 8. PMID:22316148.

[11] Iwata M, Yamamoto A, Matsuo S, Hatano G, Miyazaki M, Fukaya T, Fujiwara M, Asai Y, Suzuki S. Dynamic

Stretching Has Sustained Effects on Range of Motion and Passive Stiffness of the Hamstring Muscles. J Sports Sci Med. 2019 Feb 11;18(1):13-20. PMID: 30787647; PMCID: PMC6370952.

[12] *Growth Hormone in Aging - Endotext - NCBI Bookshelf.* https://www.ncbi.nlm.nih.gov/books/NBK279163/.

[13] Stanworth, Roger D, and T Hugh Jones. "Testosterone for the Aging Male; Current Evidence and Recommended Practice." *Clinical Interventions in Aging*, Dove Medical Press, 2008, https://www.ncbi.nlm.nih.gov/pmc/articles/PMC2544367/#:~:text=Changes%20in%20testosterone%20levels%20with,%25%E2%80%933%25%20per%20year.

[14] Curtis, Elizabeth, et al. "Determinants of Muscle and Bone Aging." *Journal of Cellular Physiology*, U.S. National Library of Medicine, Nov. 2015, https://www.ncbi.nlm.nih.gov/pmc/articles/PMC4530476/#:~:text=%E2%80%9CSarcopenia%20is%20defined%20as%20the,insulin%20resistance%2C%20and%20nutritional%20deficiencies.

[15] WL;, Westcott. "Resistance Training Is Medicine: Effects of Strength Training on Health." *Current Sports Medicine Reports*, U.S. National Library of Medicine, https://pubmed.ncbi.nlm.nih.gov/22777332/.

[16] Samson, Rachel D, and Carol A Barnes. "Impact of Aging Brain Circuits on Cognition." *The European Journal of Neuroscience*, U.S. National Library of Medicine, June

2013, https://www.ncbi.nlm.nih.gov/pmc/articles/PMC3694726/.

$30 FREE BONUSES

Get Your Bonus Exercise Companion Videos
+ Printable Workout Tracker Sheets

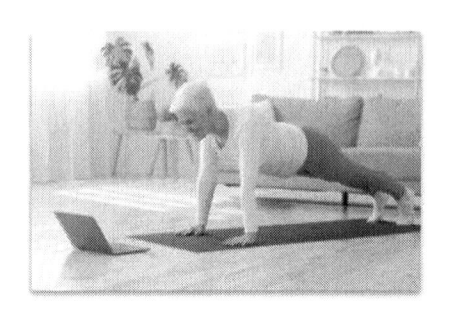

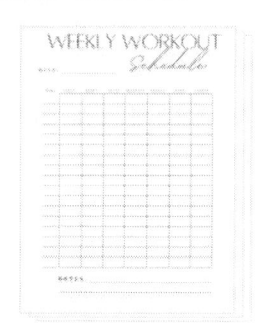

Scan QR code above to claim your free bonuses!

—— OR ——

visit https://bit.ly/3eaWvXF

Prepare to regain your rock-steady balance!

- ✓ Expert-guided exercise videos from the book so you can feel confident that you're doing them 100% right

- ✓ Tips & tricks to get the most out of your workout routines so you can reclaim your youthful strength & feel unshakeable

- ✓ Printable workout tracker sheets are included so you can guarantee that you're always progressing

Made in the USA
Coppell, TX
30 November 2022